Praise for
Out of the Gray, into the Light

Out of the Gray, into the Light proves that miracles are possible when we maintain unwavering faith and put forth extraordinary effort. This book is a must-read for every parent and any person facing seemingly insurmountable adversity as Amy shows us how we can tap into the limitless power of the human spirit that is within all of us.

—Hal Elrod, Author of *The Miracle Morning, Updated and Expanded Edition*

Story drives transformation, and this book is not only a remarkable account of Amy's journey but also a great inspiring account for each of us as we write our own story. It reminds us that, in the face of life's most challenging circumstances, the bonds of love and the strength of the human spirit can help us transform suffering into triumph and sorrow into joy.

—Dr. Jill Carnahan, MD,
Your Functional Medicine Expert*
and Bestselling Author of
Unexpected: Finding Resilience through Functional Medicine, Science, and Faith

AMY'S BOOK TAKES you on an emotional journey through the depths of adversity and the triumph of the human will. With grace, resilience, and unwavering determination, Amy chronicles the harrowing experiences she faced in her fight for survival and her unwavering commitment to stand up for her daughter.

—JUSTIN DONALD, #1 *Wall Street Journal*
and *USA Today* Bestselling Author,
Founder of The Lifestyle Investor,
Host of *The Lifestyle Investor* Podcast

OUT OF THE GRAY, into the Light by Amy D. Post is an incredibly moving account of every parent's worst nightmare and the courage to hold on to hope in the darkest moments. Amy's unwavering advocacy for her daughter's health and her determination to face her own overwhelming fears are courageous and inspiring. *Out of the Gray, into the Light* is proof of resilience. Amy's enduring love, commitment, and grit will capture readers. Her raw story reminds me how powerful our human spirit can be under the most challenging of circumstances.

—AMBER VILHAUER,
CEO of NGNG Enterprises

MY WIFE DIDN'T WANT to write this book. She dug her heels in and wanted to refuse what God was bringing her. But God knew what was best and began working in ways she hadn't expected. Writing this book was the most difficult thing she has ever done. It was a bittersweet but healing process for my wife. She needed to heal and compartmentalize what she had been through over an eight-year journey with our daughter and then fighting her own demons. She needed to forgive herself and turn thoughts of *fear* into *strength*. God knew the journey before she did. It wasn't easy. I saw my wife's highs and lows, and I knew God was working in her. She is the strongest person I have ever met, even if she doesn't think so.

—ERIC POST, Amy's husband

TAKE A JOURNEY "out of the gray" with a determined mother as she overcomes the fear and darkness of her child's diagnosis. Hope arises when the family unites by leaning "into the light" as a daughter is on the precipice of life and death. This transformational story perfectly illustrates how one's struggle strengthens a life as she preserves her daughter's life.

—DR. EDDIE WELLER,
Founder of Getting Weller,
Author, Philanthropist,
Speaker, and Entrepreneur

OUT
of the
GRAY,
into the
LIGHT

OUT
of the
GRAY,
into the
LIGHT

*A Mother Stands Up for Her Daughter
and Herself in a Fight for Survival*

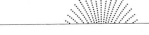

A Memoir of Advocacy and Hope

Amy D. Post

Forefront
BOOKS

Published by Forefront Books, Nashville, Tennessee.
Distributed by Simon & Schuster.

Library of Congress Control Number: 2023923591

Print ISBN: 978-1-63763-228-4
E-book ISBN: 978-1-63763-229-1

Cover Design by Bruce Gore, Gore Studio, Inc.
Interior Design by Mary Susan Oleson, Blu Design Concepts

Printed in the United States of America

To my husband, Eric

I am so thankful to be your wife.
You have stuck with me through incredibly
tough times, events that could make
the most dedicated couples waver
and hit rock bottom, not once but
too many times to count.
You continue to get back up with me—
every time—and for this I am grateful.

To my children, Zac and Madison

I am a proud mother to be able to watch
you both grow up to be strong, independent,
faith-driven young adults.
I am so proud of who you have become.
It is my privilege to be your mother.

Contents

Never fear shadows.
They simply mean
there's a light shining
somewhere nearby.

Ruth E. Renkel

A Note to the Reader

I am not a medical professional. I am—first, foremost, and for the time I am given on this Earth—a mother. When I speak in upcoming pages about the choices I've made, I am not giving medical advice. The only actual advice I offer is to love fiercely and listen closely to what God is telling you to do. Ask questions. Do research. In the end, when you come up with the direction you want to go, know that it's the one decided by *you* . . . the one that is right for you and your family. Follow your gut and don't look back; it's the only way to get through the storm.

Prologue

For a long time, I believed the best hour of the day was the one when the world was waking up. First light. The end of dark. Sun rising. Promise all around. Anything could happen in a new day.

But this daybreak was different. This one was all about choices.

Speeding from my house in the sweet suburb of Chesterfield toward St. Louis I chose not to see the sun. Instead, I chose gray. The night felt more comfortable; it was where I lived around the clock. Whether the sun was coming up or it was high noon—all I saw now was gray.

My eyes glanced at the speedometer—85 in a 60 didn't feel fast enough. I pressed my foot on the gas. In the rearview mirror I could see half my daughter's face, where she rested looking out the window. Her face was so thin the bones were like tent poles, her hair thin and fine while it grew back from chemotherapy. This wasn't what she deserved. This wasn't what any five-year-old deserved. There wasn't time to think of what I deserved, but in moments like this, the thought bubbled to the surface. Anger and desperation came at me from every angle. They weighed heavy on my heart. And so my foot turned to lead, pressing heavier and heavier on the pedal—90. 91. 92.

The other cars around us on the highway were starting to look like snails. What did those drivers know anyway? What did anyone know about us?

In the beginning, Madison and I had managed to make this drive from our house to the hospital rather peacefully, without any hint of anger or rebellion brewing. After all, I'm me—a person dedicated to making something out of nothing. The world hadn't given me much to start with, but I had made lemonade, and I had been determined to pass that trait on to my daughter.

For Madison, no afternoon was boring. She loved swinging on our swing set and the ones at nearby playgrounds. She would swing all day if she could. She loved playing dress-up. She loved singing. Dance parties. Art projects. You name it—she was busy doing it.

I made sure I lived the same way. No hour of my life needed to pass without making something a little better. Work projects, my love for my husband, Eric, time spent with my son, Zachery. If things weren't going great, the sun would eventually come out. I was sure of it. My motto was to put my chin up, work harder, pray, and wait.

Oh, but that was back in the sunshine days. Not the gray days. Not this day.

Ninety-three miles per hour.

"Mommy, are we driving too fast?"

"No, sweet girl, everything is just as it should be," I told her. But even I didn't trust the voice I heard coming out of my mouth, because I knew nothing was as it should be. After only two days home with Eric and Zac, we were going back to the hospital. Again. Maybe we would stay for four weeks, maybe more. Four weeks seemed to be the norm. The only thing I knew for sure was that it wouldn't be quick. In the last two years, we had never had an easy in and out. There had been no pleasant surprises. No day when suddenly everything just worked out in our favor.

I feel it's important to explain that so you can understand what makes a person's world go gray; what prompts a person to race down the highway, almost daring the universe to take that final step and just put us both out of all this misery; what makes a person race *toward* a place she actually wants to avoid with everything in her. If hope can't touch you, then danger can't either. Everything I believed about hard work and good people and what's fair and right had been thrown out the window. Maybe *rebellion* feels like a strange word to use, or a funny way to feel, but that day I remember rebellion seething through my system.

PROLOGUE

> *What makes a person's world go gray?*
> *What prompts a person to race down*
> *the highway, almost daring the*
> *universe to take that final step*
> *and just put us out of all this misery?*

Being told where to be and how long to stay.

Rarely being talked to, and more often, being talked at.

From the first day Madison was diagnosed with malignant liver cancer, the lack of any good reason *why*.

The gene was supposed to come from her parents, but it hadn't. Neither Eric nor I carried it.

The liver biopsy after the transplant was supposed to go off without a hitch, but it hadn't.

That morning, I could feel my foot wanting to press down even farther, but I was starting to scare myself. My car was capable of hitting 150 miles per hour, according to the odometer, but I'd never pushed it to three digits. Maybe this gray Missouri morning was going to be the one when I made it happen. What more could go wrong? Was there anything at this point that I couldn't handle?

Just one little press more, and I was up to 95. My heart started racing while I thought of Eric saying goodbye to Madison and me that morning. He knew as well as I did that we wouldn't be back for a while. Also, like me, he'd run out of words to try and make it better. I wondered sometimes if he still saw sunshine,

or if, like me, the days were mostly just gray. The old Amy definitely would have asked him that question. At the first sign of my
husband feeling down or off, I would have wanted to know what I
could do. But I was in no shape to be lifting anyone else from the
depths back to the surface—I could barely keep myself there. All
my energy was going toward keeping Madison alive.

Alive, Amy, keep her alive.

And she had been so alive. Even after the diagnosis, when
she'd started having to spend weeks in the hospital, she found so
many ways to laugh and be happy. There was the first birthday
that passed when she was sick. We were still waiting for the liver
transplant then, so I was living with a sense of anticipation, always
wondering when the phone might ring with news of the lifeline
for my little girl.

Even though she had this cancerous organ inside her, she had
spent that birthday like the princess she was. Her close group of
friends from her daycare had come to the house, all of them in pink,
lacey, costume dresses. There were games and cake, and everyone
had been smiling and laughing. I remember feeling the nerves
then, but it didn't completely eclipse the happiness. I remember
the sunshine that party day, especially when Madison laughed.
I remember one moment in particular, when she looked up and
saw her brother and dad talking to each other while they leaned
against the kitchen counter, and her smile got so big it took over
her face. That was the smile I wanted back; I wanted to see her
whole little being overcome with joy at being alive.

Alive, alive, alive, Amy. Keep her alive.

I swerved to miss a blue pickup truck that changed lanes right in front of me. I looked over, thinking I was going to give the driver a gesture like, "What are you thinking?" After all, it was daybreak in St. Louis on an average Tuesday morning; why wouldn't everyone be daring death on their way to a children's hospital?

But just then, when I was about to make my gesture, the driver of that old truck raised his hand in an apology wave. And something in me broke. I was four car lengths ahead of him in a matter of seconds, but instead of continuing to speed on, I began lifting my foot off the gas. To my surprise, as easy as it had been to press down, it felt just as easy to lift it up again.

From 98, down to 92, then under 90 . . . I watched the speed drop.

Slowly I let out my breath.

I looked at my hands on the steering wheel. They were gripped so tightly it was like I was squeezing the life out of the leather. My knuckles were way too white. I let go of my grip so I could see my hands. Fingernails I used to work to keep perfect, now half-painted and completely ignored. That was okay. I looked in the rearview so I could see Madison again. She hadn't moved her tiny face even an inch. She was still just watching the world pass by through the window. But she was breathing; she was with me. We were going to make it through the morning.

PROLOGUE

> *She was still just watching the world pass by*
> *through the window. But she was breathing;*
> *she was with me. We were*
> *going to make it through the morning.*

I felt grateful for the kind gesture of a stranger, and vowed—like the old Amy would have; some habits die hard, thankfully—that today I would also go out of my way to make a kind and unnecessary choice for someone I didn't know. As that man had shown grace, I, too, would extend an unexpected olive branch to someone. There would be plenty of opportunities, I was sure. Hospitals have a way of presenting those.

With my car back at a more normal speed, my heartbeat slowed down. After a few minutes I could hear things other than my pulse reverberating in my ears. Madison's breathing was regular and even, a picture of the warrior she had become. She'd lost that smile, but her strength had not wavered. People want to look to the parents as the sources of strength, but I knew the truth: she was the true rock here. I knew how I could show her gratitude for how hard she was fighting. It was simple, really: I would find some way to make her smile again.

Alive, alive, alive.

The exit for Children's Hospital was here, and I took it without hesitation. Muscle memory is a powerful thing, and this was the only routine she and I knew anymore.

The drive down the parkway leading to the hospital was

the only space for hesitation. That park on one side—green trees, pastures, the ice-skating rink that was just closing up after winter. Those were the things, the outdoor things, both Madison and I loved. In the great, wide outdoors was always where I had found it easiest to find God. And I needed Him now, maybe more than ever before. That was the space where I felt we needed to be, and the desire to pull the car to that side of the road was strong.

But I could see the hospital building in the distance, and we were expected to be there. As always, tests and tests had been scheduled for the day. That also meant lots of sitting would be in order. They never tell you that they schedule you for sitting, but it's the one guarantee of the hours in the day. During every hospital day.

Madison and I would sit. We would watch movies. We would look out the windows at the park and the world that we had so recently been in, which at that point would be totally out of reach. I would hold her hand and try to make her think of things she loved, but I knew the view I would have of her face would be the same one I had now. Her cheekbones. Her right eye. The perfect slice of half her nose. It was the view of her looking away, toward what she wanted to return to so badly. I didn't blame her at that moment, and I wouldn't blame her later.

I thought I heard her breath catch when I turned on the blinker for the parking garage, but it might have been my imagination. I hadn't heard that when I was racing down the highway— even her one quiet question about the car's speed hadn't contained apprehension or fear—so maybe now it was just my imagination.

If any part of me had to work to ignore the sunshine and only see gray, the parking garage at the children's hospital eliminated all that hassle for me. Cold, gray cement from floor to ceiling, winding five huge floors up—it was an *outside* view of how my *insides* felt. I'd spent the last twenty miles in feverish dismay at where we were going, but now that we were here the dismay suddenly shifted to sadness and acceptance. As I wound my way up the floors, I looked at each car, noting how many there were.

What was happening with their children? How long had they been here? What storms were swirling around them? Would they get to go home? No matter how much gray I felt inside, no matter how many more days passed before I got to see my daughter smile, I vowed I wouldn't stop wondering and feeling for these other families. They were the answers to my earlier question. Who knew what it was like to race to a children's hospital? They may not have raced like I had done that morning, but every one of them knew the desperation of having a sick child. Sadly. Heartbreakingly. Every one of them knew.

On the fourth floor I found a parking spot. I pulled in and turned the car off, and then I sat for a moment in the silence of the gray surroundings. No one else was walking around on the floor; it seemed to be just me and Madison. I looked again in the mirror at her face. The world wasn't going by anymore on the outside, but still her face was turned. When I couldn't take the silence anymore, I spoke.

"Well . . . we're here. Are you ready to get out?"

No movement. No smile.

This wasn't the Tuesday she deserved.

I wondered if I could stay in the seat and pick all the nail polish off my nails. If I should open my phone and check email. If procrastination would help her or hurt. Ultimately nothing could save us from what we had to do. The hospital doors were just across the way. Our suitcases—the ones we had stopped unpacking because we knew in just twenty-four or forty-eight hours, we would need them again—were waiting in the trunk. This time I hadn't even bothered carrying them into the house.

"I think now it's time for us to go," I said. Trying again. Doing my best at a soft voice—the voice that communicated I knew how awful this was, even though I couldn't know; I could never truly understand how difficult any of this was for her.

We might think gray is a color that covers everything—that if you are under the cloud you're just under the cloud. But she and I had been side by side for the past two years, since the day of her diagnosis. I knew all too well that the gray of her storm was different from the gray of mine. We were walking through it together, but we weren't experiencing it the same way.

I opened my car door, grabbed my purse, and got out. Then I popped the trunk and pulled out our bags. I went around to her door and slowly pulled it open. Even more slowly, I reached in to help lift her out of the seat. Whether she wanted the help or not, she didn't say. But she came with me without a fight.

I put her on her feet next to her suitcase, then I squatted

down to her level, and against the gray I was seeing and feeling, I forced a smile.

At least this time, I could speak the truth. "I love you," I told her. She didn't smile, but she heard me; I know because I saw the tiniest nod of her head.

We both put our hands on our suitcases and began to walk them in. Halfway to the doors, I started rifling through my purse, just to triple check that I had my phone. In the bottom of the bag was the desk calendar my grandma had given me twenty years before. Since she gave it to me, I had kept it close by, always careful to read the preprinted words of encouragement that headed each page. Now that the hospital was home, I took it back and forth. It reminded me of her, of strength in women, of where I came from and of what I have become, of all the places Madison might go.

The calendar had flipped open to a page in my purse. I almost had to keep myself from laughing out loud when I read the words printed there. A rebuke to my mood, a reminder that even if I couldn't feel it now, there was life outside this gray:

"Never fear shadows. They simply mean there's a light shining somewhere nearby."

With my free hand, I took Madison's and pushed through the door, wondering where that light was going to come from.

Chapter One

ONCE UPON *OUR* TIME

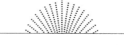

I f you told me eight years ago that every story has a very specific point at which it begins, I would have believed you. There would be no good reason for me *not* to believe you.

I've heard people tell all kinds of stories before. I've told stories. When the children were young, and I read them books, all the stories—especially the fairy tales Madison loved—had very specific points where they began. They often start with *Once upon a time.*

So I've spent the last few months going through my life, wondering where our *Once upon a time* is. I've been trying to pinpoint the one very specific point in time at which this story begins. But instead of coming up with a place where this story— Madison's story, our family's story—starts, I have ended up in the place I so often find myself these days: full of doubt. I've started to suspect that every story doesn't have an easy starting place. That not everyone has a point on the timeline where *Once upon a time* should go.

Doubt.

Full of doubt.

Doubting what so many others around me can easily believe.

If you told me eight years ago that *doubt* would ever be my go-to reaction, I never would have believed you. But I forgive that woman for her disbelief—she had no idea what she was about to live through.

You see, for most of my life, my motto was, "Life is what you make it."

I used it as a motto because I believed it was true.

When I was spending my weekdays hustling around, selling products and meeting with clients, building the work relationships that mattered so much to me, I'd tell myself that the day was whatever I wanted it to be.

If I wanted to be successful, I could make that happen.

If I wanted to double my business in a year, it was up to me to deliver.

If I was at home, picking up one of the kids after a hard fall, I would remind them (more gently) that life is what they made of it.

Would they see the glass as half empty or half full?

Would they be victims who got tested, challenged by a hill they failed to climb on a bike, or would they be victors who pushed forward and up and got back on the bike even after they fell?

Even with routine, everyday things, like conversations with Eric about what we were going to eat for dinner, *life was what we made it.*

I wanted to make life good, and almost all the time, I was successful. Life was great!

But then I got to the point where I realized that saying, "Life is what you make it," means believing that life will never throw you the kind of curveballs that can knock you down.

I watched as curveball after curveball came at us as if they were hitting each of us smack on our foreheads. They were all direct hits.

I still believe life is what you make it. In many cases, I think we can decide to look on the bright side, passionately pursue success, and become the victor. But it's not the main truth—the life motto—I live by anymore.

Now my life motto is simpler. And because it's simpler, it's easier to follow. Because it's easier to follow, it's more powerful. I think of this life motto every morning, all through every day, and before I go to bed at night. I can look anyone in the eye—even parents about to walk through the hell I walked through—and I can tell them this truth with a clean conscience, one that is not overpromising but passes along what I live by: Listen to your gut.

Listen.

To.

Your.

Gut.

My gut is what God uses every single day as a rudder to steer my ship. I don't doubt it. I don't ignore it. I learned the hard way that if you don't let the rudder move as it needs to, especially when you are in the middle of a storm, you end up in the rocks.

> *My gut is what God uses every single day as a rudder to steer my ship.*
> *I don't doubt it. I don't ignore it.*

So when people say there's one specific place to start a story, I know it would be easy to believe them. The people advising me are experts, and *whoa*, would I love to believe I can just hand some things over to experts, trust everything that comes out of their mouths, and call it a day. Isn't that the easy life? When you let experts make all the decisions about what's good and right?

But I can't. My gut says I can't do this story like other stories. My gut says I can't let the experts tell me how to write this story any more than I could let the experts tell me what was best for Madison when she was sick. (And if I had, we'd probably still be locked in that hospital.)

My gut says I can't just go through the timeline of life and find one beginning spot for the story that brought me to the low, low valley of racing along the highway, in such a dark place I did not care if I lived or died.

My gut says I can't find a place that pinpoints the beginning spot for how our family had to go separate directions for two long years. With Eric and Zac going through the motions at home, in pain because they couldn't be in two places at once, while Madison and I fought her cancer almost to the death in the hospital.

My gut says I can't locate the very simple beginning for how I decided I wasn't going to quietly file in and out of the hospital, follow all the rules, and continue doing what the doctors told me to do even as I saw it wasn't healing my daughter.

My gut says I can't pretend the storm just appeared out of the clear blue sky and suddenly began. That one day there was no rain, and the next day there was. And let's be real: if I tried to tell you that, your gut probably would tell you something was fishy. You know the weather. You understand that storm clouds brew for a long time. Even on a cloudless day at the beach, factors are mixing in the atmosphere to create an environment where a storm can occur.

Pretending there's one point where the story begins is too simple. It's simpler than our family deserves. It's simpler than you deserve. It would be too simple to be the truth.

My gut says you need to know who we were back when we thought life was only what we made it so that you can truly understand who we are now: fighters with one ear always tuned in to God.

I have one goal for putting our story into a book. By the end I want you to either know for the first time, or be reminded and reinspired, that you can live life tuned in to God as well. Calling it "your gut" is easier. "Instinct" works too.

Our lives changed in an instant when we got the diagnosis, but that wasn't the one specific point where the story began.

We just don't have that specific point in time. We do, however, have memories of a blow-up pool with a giraffe head at the front. When the pool got too full, the giraffe would spit extra water out. The kids spent hours and hours in that pool, having the time of their lives.

My gut says you need to know about those good times and that pool, what life looked like right before everything changed. So I'm going to listen to my gut and tell you more.

The giraffe pool was in the backyard at the house in Brentwood. That's how we often describe things in our family, by what house we were in when the memory happened. Maybe it's because we've only lived in two houses, so it's a very defined line in the sand.

There's the house we live in now. And then the house in Brentwood.

We left the house in Brentwood just a few months before Madison's diagnosis, so maybe that's why the house dividing line works too. The house in Brentwood is before she was sick, and the house we are in now represents a life that knows more about what can go wrong.

We can get nostalgic for memories in the Brentwood house because they were untainted and happy. I brought both my babies home to that house. Eric and I learned to be parents there. For me, the sun was always shining on the house in Brentwood. I know that's not true, but it feels that way.

When it comes to the giraffe pool though, I can be literal: the sun really was always shining on that pool.

The Brentwood house was two stories and built almost to the shape of a townhouse. Not quite as narrow, and we had a yard on all sides, but compared to the house we are in now, that house was a lot closer to our neighbors. It felt tight and cozy, and we had to make every square foot of our backyard count. Eric and I were always up for a challenge though, and we made sure that yard was a place the kids loved to play.

They were multiple ages when we lived there, but the years I remember most were when Madison was around two and Zac was about five. We had a swing set in the backyard, and there was also a rock-climbing area. It seemed like someone was always discovering a toy from the toy box that felt brand-new to them. They would get really obsessed and play with it all day long—the new favorite thing. Whenever the day was hot, the kids would come find Eric or me, begging to get in the pool, so we would put on our suits and race out to the pool.

In the house we're in now, we have an in-ground pool, which is big enough for each of us to be doing our own thing. Swimming or reading or just floating, everyone has lots of space.

But in the giraffe pool, it wasn't that way. It wasn't for adults. And when more than a few kids were in it, they were practically on top of each other. Of course, that was so much of the fun. The kids would splash around and would try to get more and more water to pour out of the giraffe's mouth. It's funny to think how Eric and I could spend so much time hanging out by that tiny pool, just watching and laughing with the kids, but we did. And we loved it.

A weekend day would often mean pool time. It would also mean the kids getting on their bikes—Madison's was so tiny and had training wheels, and Zac was just mastering his big boy bike without trainers. Then they would ride up and down the street in front of our house. They loved those bikes. I have so many pictures of the two of them on those bikes, Madison standing proudly right next to her big brother. Everything he did, she wanted to do too. She wanted to be just like him.

There was a park not far from the Brentwood house, and we would often go there. We were also lucky to have friends in the neighborhood. It was the kind of place where a lot of young families ended up. The restaurants and grocery stores were easy to get to, and it was where dusk meant listening to other families grilling in the backyard, or you would see people out for walks and jogs. And you could get to the Greater St. Louis area without too much hassle.

The day care that Zac and Madison went to was close to the house in Brentwood, and it was one of the reasons we felt that house was so right for us. What were the chances that we'd end up with such a great place for our kids to go to school just up the road?

It was a Catholic school called Carmelite. It was run by nuns who were the sweetest, most caring women we have ever met. Zac started out there, and then, as soon as Madison was old enough and ready, she joined him. One of the best parts of that school was the huge play yard that spread off the back of the property. Surrounding it were green rolling hills and huge trees, which made it feel like a magical playground was dropped in the middle of a gigantic park. The playground had several different playing areas, neatly separated by tables and benches or gardens or trees. These areas kept the playground interesting, but the kids were free to run from one area to the next. Zac would always come home with stories that included the playground. Once Madison started going there, she loved the playground as much as Zac did. She also loved getting to see him playing out there.

Because I'm in sales, I sometimes have to travel overnight. During that season in our lives, it was no different. I didn't like leaving the kids, but I very much like doing a good job for the people I work for, so when it was necessary, I'd go. During those times, I'd call home each night, and it was almost always the same story: Madison, Zac, and Eric dancing around and singing songs as loud as they could, and Zac telling me what happened on the playground at Carmelite that day.

We had everything—absolutely everything—in those

37

days. Like I said, I thought it was because we were making the best of what we had in life. Now I see it was God's grace too. A gift of happiness.

> *I'd call home each night, and it was almost*
> *always the same story: Madison, Zac,*
> *and Eric dancing around and singing songs*
> *as loud as they could, and*
> *Zac telling me what happened*
> *on the playground.*

From a giraffe pool to God's grace, that's a lot of territory, but it's what I needed to share, and I know my gut won't lead me astray. As for Eric and me, well, that story has a whole lot to do with God's grace too.

When I met Eric, I had started to think that maybe I wasn't the best at love. I'd had some toxic relationships, but nothing worth taking our precious time to recount. All of us have either been in, or known someone in, a relationship that was going nowhere, so it's pretty easy to picture what my dating life had been. There were reasons for why my relationships didn't work out: I chose someone who wasn't right for me, I worked a lot and wasn't able to invest in a relationship, I liked to do my own thing without someone getting in the way, and on and on. I'd been in love, or something I called love, but it was never an enduring love. Nothing that was going anywhere. Nothing to bet a future on.

The good news was, I had a lot going for me. I was passionate and determined; I had big goals, and I stuck to them. I was intense in everything I did and had no reason to slow down. Remember, I was making life what I wanted it to be. I moved. Forward, forward, forward.

Operating at that speed meant that from the moment I woke up in the morning, I hit the ground running. One of my friends suggested to me that if I was interested in meeting someone new to date, maybe I shouldn't always hit the ground running straight to the gym.

She said it gently, but the gist was, "No one wants to flirt at five in the morning. You're going to have to flip things around and try the gym at five p.m."

I remember thinking that I didn't want to flirt at the gym *ever*, at five a.m. *or* p.m. But I knew I did want to meet someone special, and I was working my job so much, I didn't know where else I might meet someone. So in the end, I took her advice. I flipped my schedule around and tried the gym during the five p.m. rush.

It was on one of those first days I went at that time that I noticed Eric. Boom, right away. He was there lifting weights with one of his friends. Eric looked great, of course, but that was secondary to why I was originally drawn to him. From that very first time I saw him, it was his smile. Eric's smile isn't just a smile that says he's a friendly guy. It's warm and inviting; it draws you in. It radiates kindness and safety and comfort. I don't just say that as a woman who has been married to him for fifteen-plus years; I say that as a woman who was seeing him for the first time across a gym filled with people. I felt drawn to him, wanting to feel the warmth of that comfort.

He smiled at me that first day, and I smiled back. Then the day after that. Then every day for the week after that. *Three weeks later*, we finally talked to each other. I gave him my number, and we ended up going for dinner. I won't say that I knew immediately we were going to get married and have children and spend our lives together, because my head wasn't in that space then. Back then, I thought I didn't want kids. I'd seen too much heartache up close and knew intimately how children could rip a parent's heart out. But I knew the guy sitting across from me made me feel safe and secure. That his smile lit up the room. But even more importantly, his smile lit me up. I loved being with him, so I was with him more and more and more.

There's a lot more to our story than that, but at the same time, there's not. I think maybe that's how the best love stories are supposed to be. Eric and I have always just loved being together, spending time together and hanging out. Once we got married, I thought that was it—we'd be together all the time for the rest of our lives. It was exactly what I wanted.

I had no idea that down the line we were going to be separated by sickness. When the officiant said "in sickness and in health," I always thought I was pledging my commitment to him in the worst-case scenario—if he were to get really sick. But we didn't have kids yet. We didn't know there was a scenario worse than the worst-case scenario. One when your child gets sick.

When we were in the Brentwood house, there were signs that something might have been amiss with Madison. She had been spiking random fevers for months, but the pattern was always the same. She would have a fever, so I would get concerned and take her to the doctor. Then the doctor would check her out and say it was nothing, that we should go back home and get back to making life awesome.

I didn't have any reason to disbelieve the doctors. Why would I? I'd always been a pretty healthy person and had never encountered an illness that required me to even get a second opinion from a doctor. My daughter was having random fevers. The doctor said it was nothing to be concerned about. I chose to move forward as though that answer was *the* answer.

I will tell you, though, I have regrets. Because that whole time, my gut was saying something different. After the second or third time the doctor told us to go home, that everything was fine, I felt a twinge of a mother's instinct kicking in.

Something wasn't right.

It wasn't adding up.

But the choice lay between listening to my gut or listening to the doctor. So I listened to the doctor.

Looking back, though, I'm not sure why I didn't listen to my gut. Maybe because sometimes in life, I just hadn't listened well enough.

Want to hear another time my gut spoke up and I pushed it to the side? When Eric and I were talking about moving away from Brentwood to the house we are in now, I said, completely out of the blue, "But what if something happens to the kids? This new house would be so much farther away from the children's hospital."

What? I had no reason to think one of our kids would ever go to the children's hospital! But there I was, wondering aloud to Eric about it.

He said to me, "What are you talking about?"

And then I snapped out of it. Because I didn't *know* what I was talking about. I just had this gut feeling that something was brewing, and maybe, just maybe, we would need to keep the hospitals in St. Louis within close reach. So I shook off the feeling, told Eric I didn't know what I was saying, and then we went on with our lives. Again, I wasn't a fortune teller; I was a mom. It was easy to talk myself out of why my gut feelings mattered.

We moved into the new house, unpacked our things, and loved getting to know new neighbors, new routines, new routes to school. We were going full speed ahead, with Zac and Madison leading the way.

Then one afternoon I got a phone call from school.

Mrs. Mary was Madison's teacher—and oh, did Madison love Mrs. Mary. But Mary wasn't calling with good news. She was calling to tell me that Madison was sitting down on the playground.

There's nothing necessarily wrong with sitting on a playground. I've sat down on a playground; maybe you have too. People get tired. They get worn out.

But my gut, which had been whispering to me for months was now yelling: *Alert! This isn't right! What kid just plops down in the middle of a playground? Not my daughter. She plays with her friends. She runs around. She jumps. She laughs. Every day!*

You better believe I listened. I dropped the work I was in the middle of and went straight for Madison. The whole time I was thinking, "Why would she sit? Why would she sit?"

My rational, logical side put up a fight, trying to assert it was probably no big deal and reminding me that the doctor had said everything was fine with Madison. But my gut was having none of it. Something was wrong.

As soon as I got to Carmelite and saw Madison, I could tell she was just exhausted.

I hugged her and asked what was wrong, and she said she just felt tired. Very, very tired.

> *The doctor had said everything was fine with Madison. But my gut was having none of it. Something was wrong.*

I thought that the best thing I could do was keep her in my sight, so I took her home and decided to let her rest. That way, I could observe her and see for myself if anything seemed to be wrong. Maybe we had been going too hard and pushing her too much. Maybe this was my gut saying, "Slow down the pace and be with your little girl."

So that's what we did. It was a Thursday when Mrs. Mary called, and I took Madison home. My plan was to keep her home Friday to let her rest. Monday I was scheduled to fly to California for a sales meeting, and I remember thinking we would definitely have Madison back on her feet again by then.

So all day Friday, she and I rested. And we played.

I watched her and tried to figure out if something major was happening or if this was the case of a little girl who just needed some rest.

I wish I could tell you I knew what my gut was saying that Friday, but I can't. I think about that day, and all I remember is Madison and me on the floor coloring. Red, orange, yellow, green, blue crayons. Pictures of houses. Princesses. Anything that came to mind. We colored the day away.

The resting didn't help her feel better though, and the next day she was hit with an awful stomachache and random temperature spikes. Although I didn't have a fever myself, I did have a stomachache, so Eric and I wondered if it had been something we ate.

I look back on that as one last gasp of hope. Of putting fingers in your ears and screaming so you can't hear what your gut is saying. The random fevers. The loss of energy. Now a non-stop stomachache—and not a normal, run-of-the-mill stomachache, but a bend-you-in-half pain that wouldn't let her out of its grip. This intense stomachache and a fever that shot up to 104 led Eric to take Madison to the emergency room on Sunday evening.

This is not right! Stomachaches are passing things, right? They're supposed to get better on their own.

At 5 a.m. Monday, the day I was supposed to—and was still planning to—fly to California, Eric shook me awake. He was not wearing the smile I knew and loved. In fact, it was the complete opposite—panic and fear stretched across his face.

Someone from the ER had called in the middle of the night regarding the tests they had run on Madison. Eric had taken the call, but he didn't want to wake me up then because there was nothing I could have done.

They told him that we needed to get Madison to Children's Hospital first thing in the morning. They wouldn't say why, just that she needed further tests immediately.

When I had strapped Madison into her car seat at Carmelite a few days before, I thought she would be back at school that Monday, but in actuality, she would never go back to school there. I was not going to be flying to California. Instead, I walked Zac to the school bus, careful to hide the panic that was overtaking me, and then drove to Children's, arriving just ten minutes after Eric and Madison. We were about to discover that my gut had been correct all along.

Things were not right. My baby girl was sick. Our lives were never going to be the same again.

Maybe I was wrong, maybe this is where the story should have begun all along.

Once upon a time, a beautiful, brilliant, strong princess named Madison got very, very sick.

The rest of our story is about how she fought the battle of her life to get well.

Chapter Two

JUST SOME BAD LUCK

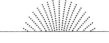

I n the terror of that first day, somehow I remember a scrap of paper in my pocket. While I walked into the hospital, looked for Eric, and was told he was already in a consulting room, I kept repeating to myself the level I parked the car on. I didn't want to forget it. Because I thought at the end of the day I would be carrying Madison back out of that hospital into the parking garage to the spot where I had parked. I thought we would be leaving.

After the nurse told me which way to walk to the consulting room, I dug in my purse for a scrap of paper and wrote "floor 4" on it. Then I put it in my pocket. I kept my attention on that scrap of paper while I walked toward the room I had been directed to. The paper was something to focus on, a reminder my car was close, and soon we would go.

Hope takes all kinds of forms—even scrappy forms.

When I walked into that stark white room and saw Eric and Madison there, I was so disoriented. Of course, I knew they would be there. But why? I couldn't wrap my head around what any of us were doing there.

I was supposed to be on a plane.

Eric was supposed to be at work.

Madison was supposed to be at school. Not in a hospital. Not in her pajamas. Not in this bland room that looked like every hospital drama I'd ever watched on television. These weren't rooms where happy things happened. This wasn't a room where good conversations take place.

As I felt panic coming on, put my thoughts back on that scrap of paper. The feeling of it. The security of it. The hope that said, "Soon you can take your daughter to floor 4 and leave."

In my wildest dreams I would not have guessed that it would be a month before we returned to my car.

This stark white consulting room ended up being a kind of home base for us to use while nurses took Madison out for tests all morning long. They would bring her back in the same pajamas . . . and a new Band-Aid. Another place she had been pricked. I could see the confusion in Madison's eyes, and I did what I could think of to comfort her.

When she was there in the room with us, I held her in my lap, feeling her body move with her breaths, trying to keep

conversations upbeat. But she knew—of course she knew—
something was terribly wrong.

When she left the room with nurses, Eric and I would just
look at each other, then at the white walls. There was so much fear
in the room that there was no space for words. When I felt myself
getting pulled under with the panic, I would put my hand in my
pocket: *Eventually we will leave, this will all be over.*

I didn't dare ask Eric if he thought there was any chance
it could be a case of appendicitis. That was the conclusion I had
come to—the "get out of jail free" card that would mean we could
return to my car, return to our new house, return to our lives that
did not know of places like children's hospitals or prick marks up
and down little girls' arms or multiple princess Band-Aids that
covered but could not cure. The way she had been bellowing over
her bellyache, it just made sense. Nothing else could make sense.
Nothing except a horrible-beyond-imagination diagnosis.

Which is what we got.

Madison was sitting in my lap when the doctor walked in
the room. I thought to myself, *Say it's appendicitis. Just say it.*

Instead, he sat down in one of the chairs by the table and
said, "I am so sorry to have to tell you this. Your daughter has
malignant liver cancer. We have to get her upstairs; her room is
ready, and her blood transfusions and chemotherapy are being
set up."

That stark white room turned black for a moment. It was
like I wasn't even sitting there. I didn't think to pray or to call out

to God; I didn't think anything at all. It was like getting hit with the full impact of a tidal wave that just knocks you out of reality. I had no words, no breath, no thoughts.

When I felt like I could see again, I was staring right at Eric. His face was such a mix of confusion, anger, and fear that my first thought was, *Go to him*. Of course, though, I couldn't. I had to go to Madison. We both had to go to Madison.

She didn't understand what the doctor had said at all, but she knew how to read Eric and me, and our reactions had scared her. Realizing that she didn't understand because she was so little just made me start to cry. Then when I tried to stop myself from crying, I just cried harder. She was *so* little. She was *too* little.

"Mommy," she whispered. "What's wrong? What's happening?"

You want to believe that in those moments you will have an answer that your child deserves. But I had nothing. I had what the doctor had told us. My lifetime of health consciousness and the security I had unknowingly found in that health shattered like broken glass right at our feet.

"We're going to go upstairs now," I told her. "We're going to talk about it when we get there."

All the time in those first months, people would tell me that "children are resilient." I was so full of anger about her sickness that I couldn't even dream of seeing any centimeter of a positive moment in her diagnosis. Now I look back on that room—that little white square that felt like it was full of the fires of hell—and

I see how Madison was the strong one. Eric and I crumbled. But all those people were right—she was resilient. When all the grown-ups were falling apart, she showed her stuff. From day one, Madison proved what she was made of.

"Okay mommy," she said, still in her pajamas. She took my hand with her little one and squeezed it. Then she told me, "Let's go upstairs and talk about it."

If I'd known anything about hospitals at the time, I would have been worried as soon as I saw we were being given a private room. This was because of the severity of Madison's condition. Stage 4 liver cancer in a three-year-old gets you your own bed and your own four walls. It gets you your own view of the park, where people run in summer and, as we would find out, skaters float along the ice in the winters.

No sharing the day with strangers. Which makes sense. What stranger could have understood what this little girl was facing? Her two parents, who loved her more than anything on earth, couldn't even understand.

Immediately the nurses started coming in and out, hooking Madison up to IVs.

I don't even know how to explain the shock of all this. My heart was back in the consulting room. Even back in the parking lot, where my car was parked, stashed with all kinds of everyday things like dry cleaner slips and empty water bottles. That life felt so different from this . . . this . . . horror movie that was suddenly playing all around us.

And not just playing around us—my daughter was playing the lead role *in* it!

The only good thing to come out of the move to a real room, the site of the IVs, and the feeling of the nurses bustling all around us was that it got me out of the make-believe stories in my head real quick. There were no more lies about appendicitis floating around. The piece of paper with the parking floor number was forgotten. We weren't getting out of this situation easily. We weren't going anywhere soon. No one had said this to us directly, but it was visible in all the IVs and machines, in the way they were telling us about schedules . . . for the next days and weeks.

There was a whiteboard on the wall. I watched as nurses went by and added their notes. Medicine names were scrawled in with the times they had been administered to Madison. Future tests were written in a different color with the time she would be taken there.

Eric and I kept looking at each other, bewildered, then at our little girl. So small. Somehow, still in those same pajamas she loved so much. I kept thinking they should switch her to a gown, that a sick patient would need a gown. Pajamas were for my healthy, vibrant Madison. The two weren't the same in my mind yet. Nothing had sunk in.

Disorientation is something we all experience. Moments in

JUST SOME BAD LUCK

life when it's hard to understand what's swirling around us. I was trying to find my bearings, but I couldn't find one central thing to hold on to.

Eric, my partner in everything, was struggling just like me.

Madison, my baby, was somehow sick with a stage 4 cancer.

Me, who always had all her ducks in a row, who was the take-charge force in the room always determined to make the most of life—who either had things under control or had a darn good plan to get them that way—didn't know where to look next.

God is where I should have gone, but I couldn't. At that moment, I just couldn't. There are all kinds of reasons I could come up with to explain why, but really, they would all boil down to one central thing: He had failed me.

Worse than that. The only thing that could be worse than that—

He had failed one of my children.

I wanted to talk to Him, but that was going to be a long conversation, a conversation I needed to think through. A conversation I needed to be present for. I wasn't ready to submit to this place He had brought us or even begin to conceive of what His larger plan might be.

Could there be a larger plan—a larger *good*—in something this awful? Even tiptoeing to the edge of that question was too much to bear.

I pulled a chair close to Madison's bed, where I could hold

her hand in mine, and I sat down. Sitting was one thing I could do.

Have you ever sat so long in the same place without moving that you wonder if you are there anymore? It's a strange feeling. Like you are both in and out of your body.

Thinking back on that afternoon in the chair, I was probably in and out of my mind.

I sat there while the flurry of activity around us continued.

I saw the first group of doctors doing their residency file in. Their leader stood at the foot of the bed facing the other residents and told them the facts of Madison's case. It felt like the man was speaking of someone else—definitely not my daughter. Spiking fevers for months. Stomachache. Blood work. The diagnosis of a stage-4 malignancy. The way he talked, it was like we weren't sitting right there. Like we were people to talk *about*, not people to talk *to*.

Without a glance in our direction or any indication we might need a little encouragement for all they'd just learned about us, they filed out.

But nurses continued to come in and out, and the beeping of the machines continued.

Madison slept a little. When she woke up, she would turn her head toward the window, looking toward the light outside, the day that was out of reach now, on the other side of the window. Time and fun that belonged to others, not her. But it didn't have her down yet, she was still smiling—the little girl trying to keep her parents encouraged.

She would turn her head toward the window,
looking toward the light outside,
the day that was out of reach now, time
and fun that belonged to others, not her.

Finally, Eric came over to where I was sitting, leaned over, and kissed me on the cheek. Someone had to leave and get Zac. We hadn't talked about who it would be; there had been no conversation, debate, or discussion. He left, and I stayed. I didn't want it any different. Looking back, I probably couldn't have been pried out of that chair. But with the countless, intense feelings flying all around, I sensed a spike of anger that he was leaving Madison and me. Just like that, he was going back out into the world, to the other side of the window, while she and I stayed on this side of the glass.

Not long after he left, the nurses' activity trickled down to nothing. Finally, Madison and I were alone.

At that point I didn't understand how hospital time worked. I didn't know that hours are counted by cups of coffee or that days and weeks run into each other. I had no idea that hours spent working for your child's smile would feel like mere seconds if she did break into a grin, but would feel like years if she didn't—or couldn't.

I thought time had stopped, and I was okay with that. Maybe if I just kept sitting, and Madison kept looking out the window, it would never start up again. We could sit in this spot of having each other, of not really having to go deep into words like *cancer* or *survival rate* or *death*.

That was wishful thinking though.

When night began to fall, a doctor came in. This wasn't a doctor I had seen before, and he wasn't one who stayed with us long. This was part of hospital time too—that different teams of doctors would mark where you were in the cycle of illness and recovery.

I knew we needed doctors, but what I needed more was an answer. I looked at this doctor, not as a man of medicine but as a human. His eyes were green, his coat was white; I wanted to believe there was kindness in his face. And I asked him the question that was foremost on my mind. After the hours of sitting, of listening, of being still while the day ran top-speed through my head, *this* was the question that was clanging like cymbals in my head.

"Why is this happening to us?"

Maybe it was the question I should have taken to God, but I still wasn't going there. I took it to this man instead. And I suffered—oh, have I suffered—for offering such a vulnerable moment to a stranger.

He put a hand on my shoulder and very calmly, very evenly said, "It's just bad luck." Then he gave me a pat, marked something on his chart, and left the room.

Good thing I was still sitting down because, when his words

hit my ears, I got dizzy and scared. Bad luck? *Bad luck?* Is that really what we were leaning on? How were we going to hope for a cure for bad luck? I mean, is a cure for bad luck even plausible?

"It's just bad luck," is what you say to someone who stubs two toes in a row. Or maybe to somebody who loses a two-buck lottery ticket.

Small things. Inconsequential things. Good luck and bad luck aren't for the big things, the life-changing things. If that's what it boils down to, then aren't we all just running around on a spinning wheel of chance? I wasn't going to believe that. Not for me, and not for my daughter.

I had the urge to punch something. And as much as I'm embarrassed to admit it, the thing that was coming to mind was that doctor's face. He was out of the room, though, and I knew I had to hold it together. I knew that successfully holding it together was the only way I was going to get through the day. (Of course, the night—when Madison went to sleep—was a different thing entirely.)

Just focus on not giving into the fear and despair lurking.

Stay very still; maybe it won't get to you.

Keep sitting without moving, and maybe more of that "bad luck" won't find you.

My urge was to find my phone and send Eric a text, to tell him what that doctor had said about bad luck. But if it had sucker-punched me, was it fair to share that with Eric at that moment? It felt like too much to put on my husband.

I couldn't help but wonder what he and Zac were up to. On that first night, the routine back at home was still so familiar to me; I could easily imagine where they were in it. I could imagine Zac's bedroom and picture him sleeping peacefully within it.

The next night and the night after that and then every other night after that, Zac and Eric came to the hospital for dinner. As would become the routine, they would sit on the foot of Madison's bed and tell us stories from the day, while Madison ate the soup Eric had cooked for her or the macaroni and cheese he had bought from her favorite restaurant. Zac would do anything to make Madison laugh. No matter how much she had been poked or prodded that day, her brother could always bring her back to a place where she was smiling. And though I didn't know it yet, I think I sensed that this was what our family did now. It was the new family thing. (What an understatement!) That first night I mourned for the normalcy that was lost. I did not want to accept that any part of this room, with the incessant beeping of machines and constant flow of medical personnel, would be our new normal.

I didn't want to accept it, but I would have no choice.

As soon as Madison started to feel sleepy, she said she wanted me to get in the bed with her. So, of course, I did. I crawled right into that space with all those cords and beeping machines, and I held my little girl. There was no sleep for me though, not even out of sheer exhaustion. Despair brings along its own kind of adrenaline; any parent with a really sick kid knows what I am talking about. This despair adrenaline shoots electric fear through your veins. That night was the first time I felt it, but it wasn't the last. Fear all around my body, pulsing through my heart. I had never feared much in my life, but I feared this.

Why Madison?

Could it really be just *bad luck*?

While the clock ticked, my mind raced—electric fear keeping me on pins and needles.

When your case is as serious as Madison's, hospital time doesn't recognize day versus night. Another group of residents came in while Madison slept. Nurses changed. The whiteboard was erased and rewritten. I lay there with Madison through all of it, just witnessing and watching, wondering what the heck my next move was going to be.

One "good" thing that happened that first night was a nurse telling me, "In the morning you have a meeting with your mentor."

A mentor? The word sounded like someone I could trust, but was there anyone in this building I could trust? I wanted to believe there was and that maybe this mentor was who I should have asked my big question to instead of the doctor.

The reality was that I desperately needed someone to talk to. Eric and I would be like the blind leading the blind; neither of us had any idea how to get oriented in this new reality. I must have dozed off at some point, and my internal alarm clock woke me at my usual time of 5 a.m. Of course, there was nothing "usual" about this morning. Even at that early hour, when I should have been in my home, with my family, waking up to have my coffee, taking our dog for a run, getting myself ready for work and the kids ready for school, I was jolted into this new reality. Strangers—nurses, residents, whoever—in our room talking about Madison with a physician. As if she were a science project! They weren't speaking *to* me or Madison. They were speaking *about* us. *Hello! We're human beings!* I wanted to scream. *My daughter is more than a diagnosis!*

> *Hello! We're human beings!*
> I wanted to scream.
> *My daughter is more than a diagnosis!*

This early-morning dream-turned-nightmare also became a routine. Every morning at 5:00 a.m. without fail—for weeks—these events played out and would continue throughout the day and evening, all the way to 11:00 p.m. Ours became a revolving door of residents, nurses, and other hospital staff barging in, many times without knocking, discussing Madison like she was a project. What an invasion of privacy! It was so wrong!

At some point, the room cleared out enough for me to feel we had a semblance of privacy. I went to the little bathroom in our room and splashed water on my face. I used the makeup bag in my purse to freshen up and then started a mental list of the things I needed Eric to bring me from home.

Deodorant will be nice.

Clean clothes.

Books for Madison.

Being able to make a list made me feel better. I realized it was the first productive thing I'd been able to do since we arrived.

I had the same clothes on from the day before—the clothes I was wearing when I was supposed to go to work, when I was supposed to bring my daughter home. I went across the hall to the small kitchen area with a refrigerator, coffee maker, and supplies. I made myself a cup of coffee. There was someone already there. The father of one of the patients, I assumed.

I had to muster enough energy to just speak, but I asked, "Why are you in here?" I couldn't help feeling like I was asking a felon why he was in the jail cell because that's exactly what it felt like. A prison sentence. And I had been here less than twenty-four hours. I was scared and confused, and I needed answers.

This was my first time meeting another parent in the hospital, and even though we didn't know each other, we immediately had the connection. He knew I was there for a reason of great sadness, and I knew the same about him before we even said a word.

While we drank our coffee, the man told me his son had been diagnosed with cancer seven years before. They had been out of the hospital for a few years, but now they were back again. This time, a brain tumor had been found. My heart fell to my feet faster than I could swallow. What could I say that didn't feel fake or false—all of us who were there knew that true consolation could only be found in healing.

He walked out of the room, and I bowed my head, tears pouring down my cheeks. I was completely humbled by his story, and I told myself I had no reason to feel sorry for myself. But only a few minutes later, I was jolted back to reality when I walked across the hall and saw Madison hooked up to hundreds of wires, and I heard beeping sounds every few seconds. My head sank to my chest again. I couldn't stay in this place . . . we didn't belong here.

Madison woke up while my head was still bowed, the tears still pouring. I quickly composed myself; I didn't want to show her my tears or my fear.

It was time for the mentor meeting, so I told Madison I would be back in about an hour. I saw the look of panic on her face, and I understood completely. So I said, "Well, maybe I won't go."

Suddenly a nurse was in the room, right behind me. She was there to support Madison. She told her that she wouldn't be far away, and if Madison needed anything, she could just hit the button. The nurse turned the TV on, and as she was putting in a movie, she slowly motioned for me to leave.

When you are in the middle of the world crashing down,

small kindnesses can feel so big. *See, I told myself, there are people you can trust here. There are people who have your back.*

I didn't realize how physically exhausted I was until I left Madison and started navigating the hallways leading to the mentor's office. When I got there, I felt I had met the person I needed to see. After being ignored, pointed at, diagnosed, shuffled around, overwhelmed, and filled with absolute despair for nearly twenty-four hours, I found the eyes I needed to look into. Eyes I could level with and ask questions of.

My mentor introduced herself, and I did the same. Then she started talking, methodically going through information, pausing every now, and making sure I was taking it all in. I knew she was trying to make it easy for me to understand, but the information made me feel like I'd been mowed over by a dump truck. I was exhausted, sleep deprived, and completely confused.

For a woman of action, a list maker, someone who thrives on doing, finding out what was going to come next was what I needed. I was still mentally in and out, I still had the huge feelings of overwhelm, but a shred of myself—the "me" I had been before all this started—was emerging.

My mentor gave me a six-inch binder of information and took me through the sections slowly. When she noticed my coffee was almost empty, she asked me if I wanted to get some more. I had the feeling that there was nothing—no amount of coffee, no sleep, nothing—that could make any of this information better.

The details were nauseating. She described how all the days, weeks, and months were going to unfold for Madison, all the chemotherapy, and then, if we were lucky, the trauma of a major, liver-transplant surgery.

To say that my head was spinning doesn't come close to conveying the extreme exhaustion, confusion, and *anger* I was feeling at that moment. Things were coming at me so fast, I couldn't think straight. I couldn't see straight.

But then she gave me the news I was certain I couldn't overcome, the truth I knew we were going to have to fight like hell against.

"Children die, Amy."

> *But then she gave me the news*
> *I was certain I couldn't overcome,*
> *the truth I knew we were going to have*
> *to fight like hell against.*
> *"Children die, Amy."*

She said it with so much sadness in her voice, like it pained her to get the words out, yet she knew I needed to know it, to *hear* it.

As I listened to her words, I couldn't even think of Madison's face. I knew associating her face with the idea of death would break me. Right then and there in that office, I would absolutely lose myself to despair.

She gave me a minute. Then she said it again. She'd done this before, and knew I needed to hear it twice for it to really resonate.

"Children die. And couples get divorced."

I thought about Eric. Eric smiling at the gym. Eric smiling when he held Zac in his arms the first time. Eric strongly and stoically waking me yesterday morning, telling me that the doctors had called in the middle of the night, and he was taking Madison to Children's Hospital.

Was that a man I could split from? Was there something that could turn us against each other and ruin the life we had built? I had never thought it possible. But now we were in unknown territory—we were facing the unthinkable.

"Amy," the mentor said. "It's not a small number of couples; 90 percent of couples get divorced."

Ninety percent.

Ninety percent.

Ninety percent.

Could it be true that only 10 percent of couples survive something like this?

Yesterday on my walk into the hospital, I saw so many parents, all of them walking with children or pushing children around in an animal-shaped cart. All of them would end up either part of the ninety or part of the ten. Eric and I would end up part of the ninety or part of the ten. That was how statistics worked, right? You ended up on one side or the other.

I thanked her for her time and left the room with my binder in hand, my head still spinning.

The night before, when the doctor had said that thing about bad luck to me, I had no idea those were words I would carry around as long as I lived. They made me mad, they charged me up, but I didn't know that they were seeding into my heart.

When that woman told me 90 percent of all couples facing this kind of illness for their child would get a divorce, I felt her words settling deep into my bones. It was like every one of my cells was listening, then wondering, then protesting. On top of the cruel unfairness of having sick children, 90 percent of the parents go on to see their marriages split apart? I knew right then and there that I would also carry those words forever. This time, I did feel them seeding into my heart.

Slowly I walked back to Madison's room. My head was spinning the whole way, and I remember how I had to put a hand on her doorway to steady myself, how I could hear the movie that the nurse had put in still playing for her. I took a deep breath while I stood there.

Children die and 90 percent of couples divorce.

I wasn't ready to talk to God, not yet. But I wasn't above begging him.

"Give us a roadmap to get through this," I whispered.

I guess it counts as prayer, but it felt more like pulling at the hems of His robe, ready to bargain with anything I had if only He could get my little girl to the other end of this cancer alive.

"I'd give up everything in my life," I told Him. "Take it all."

The job. The friends. The life I thought was so important just a day before. If He could get us through this trial alive and intact, I was ready to hand it all over.

Little did I know, He'd take me up on that offer.

Before this storm was over, my life would be unrecognizable.

Chapter Three

A RARE GENE
MAKES AN APPEARANCE

Madison and I had been in the hospital for two weeks, and I still wasn't sleeping. Her little body would fall asleep every night around the same time, and every night the routine was the same. I would crawl into bed with her, position myself next to her, then hold her until her breathing took on the regular cadence that said she was sleeping. And that's when my mind would start to race.

Once I knew she was asleep, I would slide out of the bed and into the chair in the corner. All night long, I would sit in that same post and click through websites, seeking information. Any kernel that might help my daughter was worth reaching for. If no one was offering us answers, I was going to take it on myself to find them.

I'm the first one to admit I've never been the smartest in the room. When I was growing up, I figured that out pretty quickly. Along with that realization, I also instinctively understood that this meant I would have to find another way to get ahead.

In the hospital, the same survival instincts I'd used in the real world, to figure out who I wanted to be and establish my career, took hold. I was going to find out as much as I could about the subject in front of me. I was going to learn it inside out. Then I was going to use what I learned to make a plan that would get us to a better place.

That scrappiness and fighter instinct saved me more than once—and a couple really big times early on.

I think they were staggering the bad news they gave us, which was likely wise, as people truly can only take so much. First, we got the malignant cancer diagnosis, which sent me on a research mission to learn every last thing about Madison's disease.

Then, about a week later, amid mounds of tests, blood transfusions, and beginning chemotherapy, we were told about this rare cancer gene called familial adenomatous polyposis—the FAP gene.

I felt blindsided all over again! I thought I already knew who the enemy was—the cancer—and now there was a rare gene that was part of the mix too? And this gene wasn't something we could just beat; it wasn't temporary or fleeting. On the contrary, words like *permanent* and *lifelong* were used.

I was going on no sleep, surviving around-the-clock visits from doctors and residents, digesting conversations about organ transplants, and wading through the beginnings of chemo-therapy—*and now this?* At least I knew what to do. I was going to have to research, research, research. I had my work cut out for me. The only good thing is that work is one thing I have never been scared of.

When they did the genetic testing to get to the bottom of this gene, we were going to get the information we needed, but none of it was poised to be pleasant. Was Eric the carrier? Was I? And most crucial . . . was there an unknown bomb ticking inside Zac? We had to have these answers, and I wanted them as soon as possible. In my mind, *yesterday* would have been ideal.

At the heart of the search—and at the heart of my every breath—was still this desire for a reason. Why were we here? I needed to know it was more than bad luck. I needed to know God hadn't just spun the tables on a whim—that there was something concrete we could build a defense against. I was ready to fight; I just had to know where to direct my efforts.

> *At the heart of the search—*
> *and at the heart of my every breath—*
> *was still this desire for a reason.*
> *Why were we here? I needed to know*
> *it was more than bad luck.*

That first meeting with the genetic team was in yet another white-walled room. We got information we had received before, but it wasn't coming to us second- or thirdhand. In front of us were the men and women who understood these genes, how they behaved and operated, the ways they could ruin lives.

It wasn't until Eric and I were in that room that I realized the full weight of getting these genetic tests. What if I was the one who passed this gene on to Madison, and maybe even to Zac. Would I be able to live with myself? And if it was Eric, would I be able to live with *him*? I wanted to be in a mental space beyond blame and fault. But when life and death come into the equation, you just never know how people are going to feel or behave.

I remember having the doctors repeat back to me what they'd already said—that the FAP gene was passed down to Madison from either Eric or me. And they were absolutely sure of it. I said, "It has to be in one of us," and they said, "Yes, that's how this gene works."

Eric, Zac, and I each gave the blood samples, and then it was a waiting game. I consoled myself with the fact that once the results were in, at least we would have something concrete to go on. But the waiting was difficult.

I stayed up late into the night, every night, researching. I wanted to know everything I could about what we were facing. The internet was full of rabbit holes; only one in five led somewhere that was remotely helpful. Though, in all fairness to the world wide web, my lack of sleep was likely starting to contribute to how often I felt like I'd wasted time on unhelpful sites.

Then the results came in.

As soon as they called us down to the genetic team offices to give us the results, I felt this slight tremor start in my body. I knew I was worried about the outcome, but I didn't realize how deeply that worry had entrenched itself in my system. My body wasn't going to let me lie to myself anymore though. In the elevator on the way down, I tried to steady my hand, but there was no pretending this away. I was minutes away from finding out whether Eric or I had been the one to pass down this life-threatening blow and if Zac had this in his future too.

The doctor told us the good news immediately: Zac did not have the gene!

In just a couple of weeks, I had already gotten to where I expected bad news, so I remember feeling shocked.

"He's . . . he's clear?" I asked. I just had to hear the doctor say it again, just to know for sure. And the doctor nodded his head yes.

"Now for the not-clear news," the doctor went on to say. "Neither you nor Eric passed down the gene to Madison."

Immediately my mind raced back to the confirmation this same doctor had previously given me. He said the gene had to come from one of the parents. Everything I had seen on the internet backed this up too.

The doctor was still talking: "The gene doesn't skip generations. So there's no chance of it passing over you and Eric."

"How can this be?" I asked. I remember feeling genuinely confused. I had been assured—given 100 percent certainty by doctors. At that point I still believed they were the experts and the only ones to believe, so this was truly mind blowing.

I'll give him credit, though; he didn't blow smoke or try to cover up with explanations that weren't the truth. "We have no explanation for how Madison has this gene or why the cancer developed," he said.

I sat back in that plush leather chair, letting this gray area of the unknown settle into me. I had been depending on an answer. It was the anchor I thought I'd start building from. And now . . .

"No explanation . . ." I said, trailing off. It was on the tip of my tongue, but I wouldn't let myself say it. I still wasn't going to believe it: *Guess it was just bad luck.*

If I thought I'd been researching a lot before, now I really kicked it into gear. I talked to anyone who would lend me a moment of their time—asking questions, digging in to try and get clarification. Every rabbit hole that went nowhere could, in its own way, get me closer to a search that might yield results that I needed. I refused to give up. Every time I saw my baby in that way-too-big-for-her bed, like the space was just sucking her up, I had every reason I needed to keep going.

The genetics team had also done further tests on Madison, and if their answers to us were vague, these were the exact opposite. With startling precision, they zeroed in on the cancer gene

Madison had and then predicted she would, in the course of her lifetime, endure two more cancers: colon cancer between ages thirteen and seventeen and thyroid cancer between ages forty-six and forty-seven. It was so precise, just like the first cancer Madison had: malignant liver cancer between ages three and four.

Immediately my thought was, *I'm not going to let this be her life.* I'm just not. Normally I never backed down from a fight, but I will admit, I felt my faith wavering just a bit. The precision and the knowledge they had seemed too damning. In the next breath, they said when she gets a little older, they would want to take out her eggs. The good news, they said, was that they could pluck out any eggs that carried the cancer gene and save the good eggs so Madison could one day have babies without worrying about passing it on.

The thing about good news when it's delivered with such crushing bad news is you don't register it as anything other than bad news. They believed they were speaking of possibility. All I heard was that my baby wasn't going to get out of this, ever. Even if she won this fight at age three, she'd have two more. And down the road when she wanted to have babies? She'd be reminded of it all over again.

Her life had been stripped away from her. She was just a toddler, and we were talking about her eggs! I kept thinking: *I'll take it. Give me the thyroid cancer, give me the colon cancer, I've already lived such a good life. Plus, I'm older and more equipped to fight.*

It seemed only fair! But the only thing this cancer was teaching us over and over again: fair has nothing to do with it.

Eric was in that meeting with me when they told us about Madison's cancers and Madison's eggs. He was heartbroken. I didn't need to look at him to see it—I probably couldn't have looked at him without breaking down; I could feel it radiating off him.

It was funny how, even in these unknown situations, I could still know him so well. I could sense his heartbreak when I felt his body sink as he sat in the chair next to me. I recognized the quiet desperation under the questions he would ask Madison: *How are you feeling today? What movies did you watch? Does dinner taste okay?*

In that moment with the genetics doctors, he surprised me though. His defiance came out with no warning, mixed up with his faith and, I think, with the hope he was getting every time he saw how hard Madison was fighting.

There were three of them there to tell us about Madison's projected cancers and then talk us through what we could do to prepare. Eric looked one in the eye, then the next, then the next.

Without hesitation he asked, "Do you believe in God?

The first doctor said, "No."

The next said, "I don't."

The last shook her head no.

I shouldn't have been surprised; this wasn't a place where God reigned. This was data. Science. But still, I felt something in me wilt with disappointment.

Eric wasn't giving up. "Do you believe in miracles?" he asked.

Again, they did not. One of them said, "Maybe miracles happen, but this is the data on your daughter."

My husband wasn't having it. Very quietly, but with words laced with steel, he told those doctors, "I believe in God. And I believe in miracles. I believe one is going to happen for our daughter. She is going to live."

> With words laced with steel,
> Eric told those doctors, "I believe in God.
> And I believe in miracles. I believe
> one is going to happen for our daughter.
> She is going to live."

Those doctors in the genetics office were some of the nicest we dealt with. The victory here wasn't in showing opposition to them. In the moment, I think we felt like the victory was just that we had drawn a line in the sand and said, "This is what we believe, and what we are believing for our daughter."

Looking back though, I think the victory was that Eric knew it was time to say, "We play by different rules, and there's more to this than what you can print out and put in front of us."

He had no idea how right he would be.

Even while our minds were completely consumed with Madison, trying to get to the bottom of the diagnosis and understand the big picture and, most importantly, our game plan for getting her well, the machine of everyday life was still running.

This meant we couldn't just focus on the big task at hand; other pressing needs were always appearing.

The reality of being in a hospital with such extensive care, laundry lists of prescriptions, and chemotherapy on the horizon, was that costs were going to mount up.

I know from working in the pharmaceutical world that a brief, eighteen-month dummy "script" (short for prescription) would give all the info we needed. I had to know what our prescriptions would cost us . . . could we afford them? So I went down to the pharmacy to find out. The total astounded me. I called Eric in tears, and he told me to have faith, that there was going to be a way.

That night he started a GoFundMe, and thanks to the generosity of people we knew, and a lot we didn't even know, a way was made.

It started bad but ended up good. Not just good, but great. The financial provision was needed and so appreciated, but more than that, we learned that so many people out there were rooting for us. Every time I scrolled through the list of donors, I couldn't help but tear up. People I didn't expect to know about Madison's sickness, much less donate, were giving their hard-earned money. Every day that went by, Madison and I had felt more separated from the lives we had had on the outside of the hospital. The GoFundMe was a reminder that we weren't alone. Even when we felt physically alone, we were still being backed by a whole community.

I might get hit with every GoFundMe in America now, but I'll say it anyway: You better believe that when a GoFundMe comes across my path for anyone struggling with sickness, I jump on it! The costs the health system puts on people are astounding. When most of those families are already under the emotional strain of their lives, adjusting to and then coping with a new "normal" of sickness, looming financial unknowns—will we lose the house, will we lose everything—is more than anyone should have to bear.

I know. I've been there. I've felt that load and have known how close it can take you to breaking.

While the GoFundMe reminded me there were people outside the walls who were rooting for us, I still felt a loneliness with the day in, day out of Madison's and my routine. I was inundated with research, trying to figure out how hard to push doctors, who to ask questions of—basically, how to maneuver myself around the machine that was the hospital in whatever way would be most advantageous to my daughter.

Eric tried to be there for us, but I was beginning to see a gulf spreading between us, formed simply by the separation in our roles. I couldn't put words to what it was like to be there day in, day out. I was too exhausted to try and explain to him all the details. Even when I did, I felt like he wasn't quite getting it. Then I was so heartbroken not to be with Zac—to be missing so much of my little boy's life—I knew I wasn't reacting with openness when Eric would tell me about their days.

We would have to find a way through it, I knew. But in my heart the most immediate problem was needing a confidante. Eric had been my best friend since we met, but as we were locked up in our own grief and just trying to make it through the day, we weren't there for each other in the same ways we had been before. In my mind, I heard that statistic over and over again: "90 percent of couples . . ." I knew if we were going to beat those odds, I couldn't expect him be everything in this time. We couldn't be everything for each other if we were being everything for Madison.

I still wasn't praying to God regularly. That was another relationship I was hoping would work out as time went on . . . along with a settling of my anger and frustration. When I look back now with the gift of hindsight, I am so amazed though. Even when I was turning away from Him, He never left me. He saw how alone I was and gifted me the blessing of a friend who knew exactly what I was going through, and exactly what I needed.

The first weeks after Madison's diagnosis I was emailing clients in my business as a sales rep as often as I could, literally begging them to hold on for me, to give me time to catch up with my life. "I am still there for you!" I kept assuring them. Thankfully, I had worked with everyone long enough and established enough trust that they believed me and gave me space to make good on this promise.

One day, I was making calls and ended up speaking to someone in my company. After lending an empathetic ear to all that was happening, he said, almost as an afterthought, "Do you know Kim?"

I didn't know Kim. He told me she lived two states over and was based out of another office. He had heard that she was going through something similar though. Would I want to reach out to her?

Did I want to reach out to her? I felt goosebumps on my arms—the first good goosebumps I'd had in a while. *Absolutely* I wanted to reach out to anyone who was going through something similar. The fact that she and I had the company connection made it feel even more the godsend that it was.

I reached out to Kim, and she was just as happy to hear from me as I was to hear from her. Sadly, what the man heard had been correct; she was in the same boat as me. Her daughter was older, by about ten years, and the cancer was completely different. But so much of what we were going through was exactly the same. I could have cried out of relief as I heard her talking about what worried her, what she was thinking of, all the myriad ways she was making herself sick over what was happening. I kept thinking the same thing.

Me too.

Me too.

Me too.

Never in a million years would I wish what I was going through on anyone, much less someone I ended up loving like a sister. If we both had to be walking that path though, it's the goodness of God that He brought us together.

Every night we would text for hours while our daughters slept. We were both fighting for our daughters' lives and trying to keep our heads above water. The ability to connect and to know she and I were always there for each other was something I cherished. And something I grew to rely on.

So during the day, when I was taxed or stressed about something, I would find strength to shoulder through simply because I knew I could tell Kim about it that night.

We settled into such a natural rhythm of friendship, sometimes it would shock me that we'd known each other for such a short time. And we had never even seen each other in person! If I had to list anything positive that came out of that period of time, learning how deeply nourishing and restorative friendship can be is one of them. That friendship was a gift from Kim, and God. But it wasn't just for me. It was also a gift for *Eric* and me. When I wasn't looking to him to prop me up, we had space to just stand shoulder to shoulder as we continued to wade deeper into the journey.

Madison might have been just three precious years old, but the friendship she received during that time was powerful as well. Ms. Mary's class at Carmelite kept Madison in their prayers, and they weren't going to let her forget it.

For those first weeks we were in the hospital, the class called my phone every day and left her a message. At first the sounds of all those voices lifted Madison up. Like me, she was trying to figure out what the heck was going on. How she had ended up there. More importantly, how long it was going to last.

When she asked those questions, I couldn't give her concrete answers. Like she had done on that first day in the hospital, she watched me closely. And even though I did my best to stay upbeat, the unknown of her situation likely shone through.

Her friends' voices were a balm. The connection to her school and to the life she loved with her little group of friends was strong, and when I would play the messages, it was like a cord that got strengthened. She would have me play them over and over again, then she would just giggle. It was always the same: Ms. Mary's calming voice telling her they were praying for her and describing a few of the things they had been doing, and the kids all talking loudly in the background.

The first day Madison refused to listen to the message, my already broken heart cracked some more. I had asked Madison if she was ready for the message, and she shook her head no. "Sweet girl, are you sure?" I asked. "Ms. Mary and all your friends, they left you a message to play now before we go to sleep."

She just shook her head again, then motioned for me to come up in the bed with her.

I put the phone down, thinking (and hoping) this might be a passing thing. She had been through an extra-hard day, so maybe it was that. But then the next night, when I asked if she wanted to listen to the message, she said no again. Then the night after that. And the night after that.

As the nights went on like this, it occurred to me that every last detail of Madison's body was being tracked. They had measurements upon measurements of what was going on in her physically. But beyond the physical, we couldn't know. I talked to her as much as I could. I asked questions. I loved on her. As a three-year-old, there was only so much she could communicate. If she had been thirty-three or fifty-three, with so much more living under her belt, maybe she would be able to process what was going on inside.

Again, I was struck by how cruel this sickness was. Again, it made me furious at God.

When we fell asleep at night—or I should say, when Madison fell asleep and I rested there in the bed with her, staring at the ceiling, or sliding out to research the questions banging around in my mind—it was never completely quiet in our room. Nurses came in, but they were always respectful and as quiet as could be.

Due to the severity of Madison's case, we also still had a parade of residents march through, who, unfortunately, were less respectful of a child sleeping.

Trying to keep hold of what was familiar, we tried to maintain some of the routines we had at home. After dinner Madison would brush her teeth, and we would curl up to read books and watch movies. I missed being able to put her in her favorite pajamas, but the hospital gowns were the only thing she could wear because of all the wires.

One night in the early weeks, I was curled up with her in bed, watching the ceiling and willing time to move, when all of a sudden one of the machines she was hooked up to started to go off.

I bolted upright in bed. Next to me, Madison—who must have been racked with exhaustion—barely moved, even with what sounded like a siren next to our heads. Before I could even get oriented, our room was filled with people. Nurses, perhaps even a doctor—there was so much movement I simply couldn't keep it all straight.

In the daytime hours, if an alarm like this had gone off, I would have been up and at 'em. Daytime Amy was a warrior mom, always trying to stay up with what was happening—if not a beat ahead. I asked questions. I knew what they were doing with my little girl.

But nighttime Amy had let her guard down. She had decided it was okay to take off the war paint because our routine called for it. Immediately, I saw what a mistake that was.

Everyone was in motion—they had moved me off Madison's bed, unhooked her from restrictive machines, and moved her to a gurney that was ready to roll before I could even gather myself to ask what alarm was going off. One of the nurses looked at me and asked if I was coming along. I had about two seconds to either jump on the gurney or get left behind in the room, so I jumped on with Madison.

I couldn't believe how fast everything had shifted. *Where are we going? Why did the alarm gone off? Is Madison okay?*

My panic shot up to an immeasurable level. Usually I would have been able to control it better than that, but the disorientation left my mind prone to worst-case scenarios. The staff pushed Madison and me through the hospital, efficiently opening doors and turning the gurney, using terse, quick language with each other, and I was mentally spinning. I could hardly articulate my thoughts. I felt like the opposite of what I had been striving to be since we arrived—a mom who was always informed enough and in the right place to advocate for her child's best interests.

There was a movie in the 1990s called *Pretty Woman* starring Julia Roberts. In one of the scenes, Roberts's character is upset because she has been in a situation where she feels taken advantage of. She explains that she feels like she was at a loss because she was not in her normal clothes and didn't feel like "herself"—the self that could have combatted correctly in the situation. Being out of her element had led to too much vulnerability.

That's exactly how I felt on that gurney. Without my

makeup and clothes, I wasn't ready to be at the top of my game for Madison.

When the gurney got where we were going, I jumped off, and the doctors got to work on Madison. After what felt like hours but really wasn't that long, they were able to tell that the warnings had been something of a false alarm.

That night taught me a truth that I never forgot for the rest of the time in the hospital. Never again did I completely take my makeup off, put on casual sleep clothes, or let my guard down. Madison's full-time job was getting better, and my full-time job was being ready to advocate for her.

> *Never again did I let my guard down.*
> *Madison's full-time job was getting better,*
> *and my full-time job was being*
> *ready to advocate for her.*

No alarm bell would catch me unprepared again. Day or night, I would always be ready to go. And this served me well. I came to see it was "normal" to be whisked away at a moment's notice for a procedure or to go into the PICU (Pediatric Intensive Care Unit). I had to get very good at packing up in less than three minutes. Sometimes I thought of it as some sort of military or combat experience to see how fast we could evacuate the room. Packing everything—clothes, toothbrushes, hairbrushes, shoes, blankets, stuffed animals—and throwing it all on the gurney as nurses motioned us (always prodding us to move quicker) on the way to the next destination.

Sometimes it seemed they forgot we were human and didn't understand how deeply unsettling all these crises could be. We weren't part of an experiment to see how fast people could move!

One positive about being pushed in a million different directions is that you come to truly appreciate when people slow down long enough to actually see you and your child. When there was a nurse who had a great bedside manner, we felt it. When someone slowed down to say, "I know this is hard on you; take a deep breath and then go," it was like a gift from God.

We took those gifts and clung to them with everything we had—some days and nights, that's all we had getting us through.

Chapter Four

MEMORIES BOTH
REAL AND SURREAL

I spent so much time in those weeks just watching Madison. The room was only big enough for me to have a few perches: the chair by her bed, a chair in the corner where I did my research, and then, of course, where I perched at night, curled up beside her in that hospital bed.

There were times I felt nervous to take my eyes off of her, as though by having someone watching over her, she couldn't possibly get *more* sick. I became so acquainted with her breathing, I knew it better than my own. The sound of the inhale and exhale, the rise and fall of her chest.

So often I ended up thinking about her childhood. The one I wanted for her . . . and how far away that vision was from what she was actually living. I became acutely aware, in a way I'd never been before, what a precious gift those young years in life are. Only when I saw the carefree innocence robbed from her did I realize how much it had meant to me. It made me look at my own growing up years and wonder how the threads of those years tied to the woman and mother I am today.

As an adult, I can look at my parents' relationship—they are still married but live separately—and I think their relations when I was a young girl were probably strained. As I got older, in my teenage years especially, I saw signs of that. As a very young girl though, I either didn't see signs of strain, or I just looked past them. My very young childhood came with a freedom I've never known again as an adult. But it set the bar for a level of everyday happiness that I am so grateful for. I truly believe that freedom gave me the fundamental belief that life can be what we make it.

My mother worked in family services, and she was a hard worker, both at her job and at home. She was selfless with her time, working all week from 8 to 5, commuting a fairly long distance, and then giving up her weekends to clean the house and prepare meals for us for the coming week. It was important to her to take care of all of us and to pay the bills. She certainly delivered on the work ethic that said, "Nothing is handed to you. If you want something done, do it yourself."

My dad was the opposite. He bounced around. If it was a new year, he was probably doing a different job. He was very handsome and had a great voice. Because of these traits, there was a lot of work for him at radio stations and as a model. In addition to having the "right look" to be a model, he was also a professional water skier and scuba diver.

It's no surprise then that my dad was a great lover of the

outdoors. My mom had grown up on a dairy farm and was very used to life outside a city. So when Dad suggested life in a cabin in Colorado, that was fine with Mom.

My memories of living in Meeker, Colorado, are some of the most vivid memories I have. Our log cabin had a beautiful yard, with pine trees filling the yard on three sides. My brother and I spent hours running, playing, and riding our bikes until sunset. We also played for hours with our small box cars in the dirt piles our father built for us. This is where my love for nature, and especially the mountains, began. Each weekend we would go horseback riding, and in the winter, my father would ride the snowmobile while my brother and I skied behind, laughing and carrying on for hours.

Life was good. Actually, life seemed amazing! Maybe I remember these days the best because I didn't have a care in the world. The outdoors has always offered something to me that nothing else in this world could—peace, serenity, and calm—intangibles that I value so much. My parents owned a radio station, and I would spend time with them there. I can close my eyes and remember walking down the large staircases in my parents' radio station, to the crosswalk, and across the street to the corn dog stand. I would have a few dollars each day to grab lunch. I would walk back across the street and up the multiple staircases to enjoy my favorite lunch. It's weird now, looking back, that I was three and four years old, and my parents let me do this. Was it because I was mature enough? I don't know, but my father would tell me later they can't believe they allowed me to do this. I guess they never had to worry.

At home, Chad and I had that same kind of freedom. Our playtime was always innocent and close to idyllic—lots of bike riding and just playing in the great outdoors. We would often take four-wheelers to the creek; my dad also had motorcycles around—gigantic garages filled with man-sized toys.

> *The outdoors has always offered something*
> *to me that nothing else in this world could—*
> *peace, serenity, and calm—intangibles*
> *that I value so much.*

One memory from those early years that wasn't positive, though, was when my appendix almost burst. When I was three years old, I spiked a fever and was rushed to the hospital. It is such a vivid memory and also a foreshadowing of my brother's and my future relationship. It happened on his fifth birthday. My appendix had almost burst, and I was minutes away from a serious situation and possibly even death, yet the attitude was that I had ruined Chad's birthday. And he wouldn't let me live it down for over thirty years. Maybe his teasing was tongue-in-cheek, but I have always sensed the absence of gratefulness on his part that I was okay. I realized later that my brother had always been a bit selfish, but at the time, I didn't want to see it. He was my big brother and my best friend.

I have sometimes wondered if my own experience with appendicitis is what gave me such a strong feeling—and hope—that Madison's stomachache was also tied to a problem with her appendix. It's funny how our minds work, making connections between haphazard and unrelated things. Sometimes it works in our favor. Not always, but sometimes.

During the school year, Chad and I rode the bus to school. My favorite part of the day used to be the walk from our bus stop to our front door. Chad and I would talk about our day and laugh. As soon as he and I were back by the cabin and he was joking around and telling stories from the day, it felt like school was a million miles away.

Learning was always so easy for Chad. He never had to spend time worrying about getting things done in school. Not only was he smart, but everybody at school also felt the same way that I did about him. He had the same easy charisma that my dad had, where people just gravitated to him. And whatever he was doing, they wanted to be doing it too.

When I was five years old, we moved out of the Colorado cabin and on to Taneyville, Missouri, which was even smaller than Meeker. My mom wanted to be closer to her job. And then, when I was in fifth grade, we moved to Ozark, an hour away from Taneyville. I suppose life had to go on, and that simple time in Colorado couldn't have lasted forever, but I do look back on it with a lot of fondness. It feels like a blip of undisturbed freedom I was lucky enough to experience.

When I look back on those happier years, I can still see a gap in our lives—we never had a regular church experience. Some people might not think of this as a gap, and when I was little, it didn't bother me too much. But as I got older, I found myself really wishing we had that sense of community that you can get from a church. Whenever we tried a new church, it would always be the same story. We'd go in, and my mom would quietly cry through the service.

As a kid, I thought that was just what my mom did. I didn't question it too much. And she wouldn't open up to me even when I did ask. Now it makes me really sad to consider what she must have been dealing with. Getting to know my mother has always been difficult. I didn't want it to be this way; it just was.

So every time we tried a new church, or even one we had tried before, Mom cried. It was as if she wouldn't want to go back and deal with that again. I can't blame her, but I do wish, for her sake, she'd tried to press in harder to figure out the source of that unhappiness. For her to get through it, she would have had to do a total surrender—get down on her knees and give it all to God. I think that was too much to consider.

Looking back, I wonder if a church could have made a difference with where our family went next. There's no rewriting history, but it's impossible to examine the big picture without wishing something had intervened and changed where we were going.

The differences with Chad started around the time he turned sixteen. It was subtle at first; I only noticed because I was so attuned to him.

As soon as he had his birthday, he got his driver's license and his own truck. Music was important to him, so his stereo system and speakers were in the middle of the front seat of that pickup. He took me to school every day, along with at least one or two of his friends, so I always ended up being the one who had to sit in the middle on top of the woofer. I remember driving through town with that bass rumbling. Every time the song got really loud, my seat—and then *me*—would literally shake.

Over the course of a couple months, I started noticing that Chad was more distracted, less interested in what was going on with me. We were joking around a lot less. He was talking to me less too.

Soon, I started to see physical differences. His skin looked really different, kind of dry and sunken. And his teeth were becoming discolored. I guess somebody on the outside could have written the changes off to adolescence, but I had a gut feeling it was something different. His attitude wasn't just distracted at that point; he got to where he was completely checked out, and he just didn't want to mess with me or the family at all. And if he did involve us, it was so he had someone to direct his anger and hatred toward. There were nights he wouldn't come home. It was the time before cell phones, so we had no way to track him down. We'd just wait. And pray.

Chad had some really good friends. I knew the ones who had been around for a long time. But there were new people he was hanging out with now, and I didn't know them. One of Chad's friends, someone I knew pretty well, came to me one day and said he wanted to talk. He told me he wasn't going to be involved with Chad anymore. When I pressed him, he finally told me why; it's what I had already suspected: Chad had gotten pretty deep into drugs.

I'd been watching my parents live in denial; they refused to act like anything had changed with Chad. They stayed stoic no matter what antics he was up to or whether he was paying attention to us that week or not. I assumed their denial would only go so far, though. Surely if confronted with information like this, they would want to . . . to do something.

Never in a million years would I have guessed how wrong I was.

The day I finally got up the courage to tell them what Chad's friend had told me, I waited until the three of us were together in the living room.

My mom loves bunnies, and she had a collection of ceramic bunnies that were always dressed up in costumes. She kept them everywhere—all through the house. But I especially remember them in the living room that day. Maybe because it felt like such a monumental conversation we were having, and those bunnies were the only "witnesses" to the insanity that was unfolding. The bunnies saw me tell my parents that Chad was using drugs. The bunnies saw my parents completely deny that it could be possible. They saw me try and try to convince them of the truth. Then the bunnies heard my parents say, "How dare you say something like that about him?"

It would be their stance for years and years to come.

To them, Chad was in the right, no matter what. And that meant I was in the wrong.

I was heartbroken. There I was, on the cusp of turning sixteen, going to my parents with what I knew was the truth about my brother, and they were refusing to listen. If they wouldn't believe the truth, how would we help Chad? And Chad really needed help. In that moment in the living room, with those bunnies positioned around us, and my parents looking at me with absolute disdain, I felt so misunderstood. And helpless.

And so alone.

I was heartbroken. There I was, on the cusp of turning sixteen, going to my parents with what I knew was the truth, and they were refusing to listen.

I have often thought of that time and the promise I made to myself that I would never in my life make anyone feel as alone as I felt right then.

It's easy to think of how ties connect the happy parts of our lives to each other. It's harder, though, to think of how the hard times and great losses we endure are also tied together. But when I think of how I immediately snapped to action to help Madison and how her diagnosis made me want to fight to the very last breath, it takes me back to that moment in the living room. I had felt so unable to fight for my brother, who was also my best friend. It was also the moment that I felt Chad spin further and further away from me.

I wasn't going to lose another person I loved—I just wasn't. No matter what it took, I was going to make sure Madison made it through.

Chapter Five

QUICK DECISIONS
AND BEING VOCAL

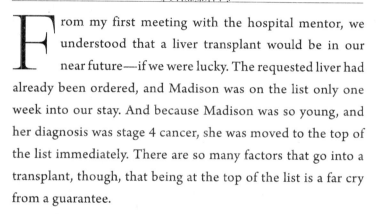

From my first meeting with the hospital mentor, we understood that a liver transplant would be in our near future—if we were lucky. The requested liver had already been ordered, and Madison was on the list only one week into our stay. And because Madison was so young, and her diagnosis was stage 4 cancer, she was moved to the top of the list immediately. There are so many factors that go into a transplant, though, that being at the top of the list is a far cry from a guarantee.

The nerve-racking thing was that there simply was no way to know when it might happen! So as soon as we were on the list, we knew there was a chance we could get the call at any moment. Maybe tomorrow, maybe nine months from now. It truly was a waiting game—and a worrisome one at that.

While we waited, my main charge was the research I was doing. I wanted to learn every last thing about possible paths to healing for Madison, and part of that meant implementing what I was learning.

I didn't have to dig very deep on the internet to find people saying the better a patient's overall health, the better they would be able to fight cancer. It just makes sense, doesn't it? You need your body to be as strong as it can be. One of the main ways someone can make sure they are operating at their optimum levels is if they are getting optimum nutrition. The first and most obvious thing I targeted was what Madison was eating in the hospital. Immediately, I started paying attention to her meals.

I was shocked at what was coming into her room on the food trays! I'm no nutritionist, but I could see it was the opposite of anything we ate at home. Breakfast had lots of muffins, pastries, fried foods, and things I couldn't recognize. Lunch and dinner would be pizza, fried chicken, or hamburgers. Those are foods many people love but that our family has never eaten regularly. When Madison was in need of healthy food to help her body grow stronger, these were not foods I would have chosen to feed her. If she didn't eat this way at home, why would we start eating like this here—a place where she was supposed to get better so she could *go home*?

I wanted Madison to have the best fighting chance, so I couldn't help wondering why a hospital, the place where people go to get well, would be serving food that would bring their health down.

I started to wonder if these foods had always been served or if healthier foods had been served in the past. Why on earth would healthier foods be promoted outside hospitals for the general population but not inside hospitals where people who were sick needed to get well? I wondered about the food choices for the health professionals as well. The doctors and nurses who were working twelve-plus shifts, six or more days per week. They needed good food for their engines to keep going. I wasn't okay with any of this, and the more questions I asked, the less okay I was with the answers. I felt the fighter in me coming to life and knew that until I got healthier food on Madison's tray I wasn't going to back down.

Getting to the bottom of the food choices offered is when I really started getting the chops to know how to fight for Madison. I wish there was some way to turn it into a formula or a bunch of steps that would explain how I went about getting changes for my daughter—so often when I talk to people about our experience, that's what they want to know. But there's just no way to narrow it down to a handbook-type setup for people, and honestly, I would question anyone who said they could!

> *Getting to the bottom of the*
> *food choices offered is when*
> *I really started getting the chops*
> *to know how to fight for Madison.*

When it came to the hospital food, I started kindly asking questions of the people who delivered it: "Is this a typical meal here?" "When was the last time they served vegetables and fruit?" "How does the menu get decided here?" "How long has that person been in charge?"

My strategy wasn't to go in with guns blazing. I was more focused on getting the big picture so I could understand what I was working with.

My friend Kim, who was living a parallel path to my own, just at a distance, completely understood this approach. Every night when we debriefed, I would tell her how Madison was doing, what tests had revealed, or how her chemotherapy was. Then I would tell her what I had learned that day about the food or the FAP gene.

Part of why these conversations were so helpful to me is just the nature of friendship, plain and simple. When we have people who care for us and listen to us, we are strengthened to go on. I know that. But I think it was also because she was seeing a similar reality unfolding around her. Like me, she was trying to figure out how to make progress in a system that appeared dead-set on keeping you locked right where they wanted you. She knew that answers to questions weren't just answers, that sometimes they were ideas being stirred and nourished so that a plan could grow.

Eric didn't understand my approach quite as well. We didn't have direct conflict about all the research I was doing or the fact that I was beginning to raise my hand and ask *why* a lot more. But I felt a low-level stress building between us.

After a few weeks, the doctors felt that Madison was stable enough to go home—not permanently and not for any set amount of time. We could take her home as long as we were ready to come back immediately if her care team found something iffy in her bloodwork and felt like she needed monitoring. Unfortunately, this happened so often that we were never home for more than twenty-four to forty-eight hours at a time during those first several months.

The first weekend Madison and I were able to go home, Eric and I finally discussed some of this stress. What should have been a happy occasion turned into an especially hard weekend. For weeks I had been in a constant state of overexertion, confusion, sadness, disorientation, exhaustion, on and on. I was in a mind frame unlike any I had been in at any other point in my life—I literally staggered into the house in need of any rest I could get. Unfortunately, it didn't end up being a time of rest.

Eric's family was in town to see Eric and to visit Madison. The weekend was a blur, but I do remember when the conversation turned to Madison's care, I discovered no one was on board with how I was approaching some of the situations: her doctors, the food, all the things I was bumping up against and starting to ask questions about. I was making too many waves, causing too big of a fuss; they were concerned that pushback toward "the way things were done" would prove unhelpful—or even destructive—to Madison's care.

Everyone there wanted the best for Madison, which

bonded all of us together. But there was no getting around the fact that we had very different definitions of how "the best" would be achieved.

And then someone said the words that still echo in my head: "If you keep talking, people won't like you."

My jaw dropped when those words were spoken. *I don't care if people like me! I care about my daughter getting better!* Yet I tried to give them the benefit of the doubt and thought that maybe I heard it all wrong. But there was no mistake. The family's desire was that I cease and desist from not only asking questions but also pushing for answers to those questions about some of the practices in the hospital system.

Was this really how my family felt about my fighting for Madison? My mind swirled through all the emotions. The confusion and disorientation that were already a regular part of my days were now amplified, but they were so much worse because the source had shifted from the inside—from our family, where I thought I could rest.

It didn't take long, though, for that confusion to turn to anger. These voices were finally putting words to the tension I had only been feeling. I wasn't imagining it. But they weren't in the hospital day in, day out. They weren't having to wake up to and go to sleep in sheer hell. All the questions about what our future would hold . . . It wasn't the reality they were going to sleep and waking up to every single day. Couldn't they just support me and trust in what I thought was best?

These emotions weren't what I wanted in my home, the place where I had been looking forward to returning *and retreating* for so long! They mixed together like a dangerous cocktail of defeat. That day, I felt just as I had so many decades before, when I had tried to help Chad by telling my parents about the drugs and they rejected my efforts. Once again, I felt like I was at fault for being myself and doing my best to care for someone I loved.

> *Once again, I felt like I was at fault for being myself and doing my best to care for someone I loved.*

It's one thing not to have the support of the world— nobody would even *expect* that. But to not have the support of your family? It's devastating. I told myself then and I tell myself now that it doesn't matter, that I can do anything on my own. But when life presents these moments of feeling separated from the people who really matter to me, it's devastating for me.

I had to make a decision though. I had to decide if I was going to change how I responded to situations regarding Madison's care because of what others thought about me. Even if they were people whom I loved dearly. It was a clear choice for me to make. Madison came first. I would not stop fighting for her.

After one of the last "big" conversations of that weekend, I went to Eric's and my room for some alone time. I had so many feelings and thoughts bouncing around. Thankfully, even with so much tension and stress going on in the background, I stayed balanced enough to ask God if I was on the right course. (He and I had begun talking again.) It's important not just to stay true to myself, but to stay true to what He wants for me. It's a key distinction yet a crucial one.

At the end of that time and conversation with God I felt like I was on the right path. I was going to fight the way I knew best, even if it meant standing alone. I was hurt, but I was no longer defeated. I didn't want anyone to be upset with me. But at the end of the day, I was the one at the hospital. And I had to try and work the system to benefit Madison. I took the cocktail of defeat, poured it down the drain, and recentered myself on the task at hand—the task that mattered more than any of our adult opinions, feelings, or plans—I had to get my sweet girl well again.

When I got back to the hospital after less than a weekend away, I scheduled more meetings with hospital management about the food, and I kept on with one conversation after another with the goal of getting healthier food options for Madison. Eventually, we began to see progress. The menus didn't change for everyone, which I then had major concerns about (and still do to this day), but Madison's trays started coming in with more fruits and vegetables. I started to see more of a balance in what she was served. Some days they were only small changes, but seeing them really mattered to me. Someone else may not interpret it this way, but I felt like it was God showing me that speaking up had been the right thing to do.

106

Each day I would tell the nutritionist or the nurses what I wanted them to order from the store, and it would be delivered and prepared. The food was still a far cry from what I would have made Madison if we were at home, but the determination and perseverance did help us make headway! This positive progress showed I didn't have to have a huge cadre of people supporting me. It didn't matter if I was one woman alone making waves, nor did it matter what anyone else thought about those waves. If I saw changes in how Madison was treated, that's all that mattered. It's what all this was about.

Even with these improvements, the biggest issue, which was always hanging over our heads, was the transplant. We were at the top of the list for a new liver, and it was the only way we were going to be able to get out of that hospital for good.

Every day there was a chance we could get called, and when we did, Madison had to be ready for a surgery. It was a responsibility that such a little body should never have to take. That little girl needed all my attention, and I was determined not to be distracted.

Yet, I continue to feel the tension, along with the deep question of how I was going to be able to keep this pace while still carrying my responsibilities: work, communicating Madison's care with the family, raising money, researching, and above all, trying to hold myself together.

I had been telling myself I was ready for the call. Any moment, I was ready. Yet when I finally got the call, and we were told we had the chance at a liver, I discovered I was totally and completely unprepared.

I should have wrapped my head around it sooner, but I had avoided the most obvious part of a transplant: for Madison to get a liver, someone had to die. It's a very basic, but heartbreakingly difficult, truth to accept.

They told me it was a pediatric liver. When I heard that, my heart dropped faster and farther than I knew was possible. The idea of those other parents out there grieving at the very minute I was receiving the "good" news we had been waiting and praying for . . . One thing about disease and sickness is that they continually provide proof that this world is not fair.

Time is of the essence in all transplants, so there wasn't much time to decide if we would accept this liver. But that was okay. I was the only one at the hospital with Madison, and Eric and I had already discussed what our decision would be. So I didn't need the time. If a healthy liver was available, and the doctors were recommending it, we wanted it.

I told them we would take it.

The doctors had been very clear with us about Madison's situation. The reason she had been in so much pain that day on the playground at school, the weekend following, plus all the days since, was the state of her liver. The malignancy was causing it to expand in her body and push against other organs, which was causing her great pain. And even though the cancer had not spread from the liver to other parts of her body at that point, absolutely no one could guarantee that as time went on, it wouldn't happen. As long as the liver was in her body, cancer spreading was a looming threat.

There were no two ways about it: the liver had to go.

Immediately after I told the doctors we wanted the liver, I called Eric. "It's time for the transplant," I told him. No more conversation was necessary; he said he was on his way.

Once the wheels for a transplant are in motion there are a thousand little pieces that have to line up perfectly before it's a "go." All of Madison's levels were already being monitored, but all this monitoring would now be under a microscope. Her body had to be at just the right balance to be optimized for accepting a new organ.

Eric arrived with dinner, and after we ate, the team prepped Madison for the surgery. I had such a mix of apprehension about the upcoming surgery, a heavy sorrow for the unknown family who had lost the child, and then the guilt that we would benefit from their loss. Part of me wondered if we could really be so close to the finish line. In this race, which had been nothing but grim difficulty, was there actually going to be a win?

My answer came at 6 a.m. As was the way of the hospital, we had spent hours and hours waiting only to find out in a short, quick burst of information that everything had changed. And not for the better. A doctor came in and told us the surgery was off.

Madison's blood work had come back, and some of her levels had spiked, indicating that if she were to undergo surgery, her body would not accept the liver. They were going to move down the list and give it to the next candidate.

"You'll go back on the list, at the top," the doctor told us.

We told him we understood and thanked him, but I was telling a lie. Really, I didn't feel thankful at all. We needed a break, and soon.

How much can one child bear? That's the question that kept running through my mind. I hated that everywhere I turned in that hospital—whether I was walking through the halls or playing with Madison in the playroom or taking her up to the garden on the roof—I saw so many tiny, precious kiddos who were all answering that question. All of them were carrying loads heavier than they deserved.

Behind them were parents, doing their best not to break in the middle of this broken hospital system in this very broken world.

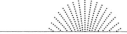

The weekend after the first liver transplant fell through, we were able to go home again, but just for a quick turnaround to get clothes and to sleep one night. When we were there, Madison still opted to sleep with me. Since the night of her diagnosis, we hadn't spent a night apart.

That Friday, I was sitting on the couch, doing some work when my phone rang with the hospital number. I don't know how I knew what the call was about, but I did. Before I answered the phone, I knew what they were going to say: they had another liver.

This time it wasn't such an easy yes though. This liver wasn't cut and dry. It came from a donor who was in the prison system, so his liver was high-risk. He was in his twenties and had died from some kind of trauma. Again, my heart went out to that man, his family, and the people who loved him, and for how life can get twisted and turned and fall away from us.

I had a decision to make. In that moment on the phone, I had to tell them if we would accept the organ or not. If my answer was no, it would be offered to the next candidate on the long list of people who needed the organ just as badly as Madison did.

This experience, and the stress of it, was magnified, but it wasn't foreign. I'd been making decisions like this for Madison, for what felt like every hour, since she'd been checked into the hospital two and a half months before. Life in the hospital was full of contradictions like this—where the pace feels like a slow crawl yet punctuated by decisions that have to be made in an instant. When those decisions come up, it's more daunting and much, much scarier than I'd like to admit. These are life and death decisions, and there's no way to make them and know 100 percent you are going the right way. My biggest fear in my entire life has been—and still is—if I am making the right decision for Madison.

OUT OF THE GRAY, INTO THE LIGHT

I sat there on the couch wrestling and hurriedly praying, trying to discern what God wanted for Madison. Was this the right liver?

That's how all those quick decisions were. In those life-threatening situations, we can be selfish without realizing it. We pray and beg and make promises for things we can't even fully understand or know. I would have promised anything, wagered anything, sacrificed anything. Part of that is what being in the hospital does to your mind. You're completely restricted, almost like a test to see when—not *if*—you break.

I couldn't allow this phone call to be where I finally cracked though. This decision had to be made, and it had to be made with my heart, mind, soul, and body. There wasn't time for me to call Eric; they were insistent that there simply wasn't time. I understood the timing, of course. The organs have to be transported and kept cool, and in this situation, it wasn't just the hospital imposing something on us, but the prison system too. This truly was the timetable for keeping this liver in good shape for whoever was going to get it.

Once again, it was all on me to answer this heart-wrenching question.

Just thinking about the list of people who wanted this liver was so difficult. Knowing we weren't alone on this gruesome path offered some comfort, but it was also bittersweet. How could I weigh all these factors? Slowly and carefully the person at the hospital explained the details about this particular organ. Because it was an adult liver, it would be portioned for two pediatric

112

patients, and each would get one bile duct. Would its "high-risk" label come back to haunt us? How could I know?

I accepted the liver for Madison, but I asked if I could speak with the transplant surgeon. I had to leave a message with his answering service, but he called me back within minutes! I just had to know something: "If it were your child," I asked him, "would you take this liver?"

He was the right person to have talked to. "I've looked at this liver, and it's a good liver," he told me. "If it were my child, I would take it."

I was ready to do whatever he said after that quick call. It's just another characteristic of being in the hospital system; you get so used to being treated like the last one who needs to know, that when someone prioritizes you, it feels close to a miracle.

Without the approval from the surgeon, I'm not sure I would have felt comfortable with my answer. There was no escaping the fact that we had a small window of time, and both Eric and I had felt more and more like our backs were up against the wall. I felt pulled in a million directions every day—missing Zac so much, and hating that we weren't together, yet knowing I was the only one who was in the position to support Madison like she needed. Until she was ready to go home, I wouldn't be able to see him anymore. Then there was my need to advocate for her and to learn how to do that, yet I didn't want to alienate the family Madison and I so desperately needed support from.

The only way out was a full recovery—it was the only

option I was allowing in our field of vision. For that to happen, we needed the liver. I wanted more than twenty-four hours at home, but I was used to this routine of getting back to the hospital quickly, and I had come to the realization that my life and Madison's life didn't belong to us any longer. We had to stay positive. I was absolutely sure that staying positive was the one thing that could help her in this surgery. So I packed up my and Madison's things. We had one hour to get back to the hospital so Madison could be prepped once again.

> *I was used to this routine*
> *of getting back to the hospital quickly,*
> *and I had come to*
> *the realization that my life*
> *and Madison's life didn't belong*
> *to us any longer.*

As we walked in the doors of the hospital, I had to remind myself that, at the end of this trip, we might actually have a new liver in Madison. I still wasn't holding out hope. I was prepared for the worst, that it wouldn't work out. And of course, the thought that she had the rare FAP cancer gene crept into my mind more than I liked. I had to try and focus on one thing at a time though—easier said than done for someone who juggles and schedules all day every day. My brain was primed to worry about a million things at once, but I couldn't give into that. I had to focus more than I ever had before; I had to find calm and get us through the battle we were facing at that moment.

Madison and I talked of a positive surgery, how it was going to be hard but that she was a fighter, and this was how she was going to fight. I remember how sure she was that this liver was going to work out, how there was no doubt that she could make it through the surgery and recover.

Inside I was full of such fear and doubt though. Here we were, going in for a second time. It was the second chance at the liver I had wanted so badly. Would it work this time? Would we ever get out of here? I prayed that God would show me where I needed to place my mind. I needed Him more than ever. I wasn't sure if my conversations with God would turn out well, but I needed a conversation with Him, whether positive or negative, to set the record straight. I needed my daughter to come through this. I couldn't live without her, and neither could her dad or brother . . . this simply wasn't something God could get wrong . . . so there again, I was asking for miracles and favors: *Lord, how do I pray correctly? How do I ask correctly without sounding so selfish?*

Once again, I was in awe of my four-year-old. How much stronger she was than me, how when times were really tough God was using her as my compass and true north.

What Madison believed was true. The hospital ran the same battery of tests, and every one of them came back perfect. Her body was in sync. Her levels were primed. When surgery time came, she was ready.

Eric and Zac came up for dinner that evening prior to the surgery, and I have never been so glad to see anyone in my life, especially Eric. Madison was in her Disney pajamas she loved so much. We ate dinner together in the small hospital room. We laughed and tried to keep the conversation light. God knew what we were all thinking; we were all so scared. I'm glad, though, that God didn't reveal any of those details to us because I'm not sure I could have made it without melting into the floor at a moment's notice. My fear was getting the best of me. How wouldn't it get the best of anyone in that situation?

The transplant day was an out-of-body experience. It reminded me of the day we found out how sick she was when I wasn't really "there" in the room. The day of her diagnosis I had been out of my mind with grief, and for the duration of this day I was lifted to a place of serenity.

No one can predict exactly when the liver will be ready. So much has to happen to properly transport and prep the organ. I stayed with Madison as long as they would let me, and then there was the point where they told us we had to say goodbye. What calmness I had came from God; there was no other source, no other way that I was able to smile at Madison and walk out of that room, holding her sure belief in a successful surgery. No two ways about it—that was grace.

The surgery was predicted to be about ten hours. Ten hours is a long time to sit and wait on anything, but I can assure you, when you are sitting and waiting on your child to get through a surgery, it's even longer. Again, by God's grace, it passed without major difficulty.

Eric, his parents, and I were in the waiting room. They somehow knew—I believe God gave them the intuition—that I needed space. Without my saying a word, they let me be alone. And for most of those ten hours, I sat in a chair with a novel, just reading and praying and being very, very quiet. She was so little, but we were told that would play to her benefit. Time and again, doctors saw how the youngest were the most resilient for liver transplants. Success rates were high. The statistics on young bodies accepting the livers were high.

Looking back, I can't believe how much peace was flowing through me. Just a couple of weeks before, there was one night when I had lost it. Madison had been asleep, and one of the nurses I knew well and trusted came into the room. She was whispering to me, checking on me, making sure I was okay. Out of nowhere I started crying. I'm sure she had places to be, but that woman just stayed there, letting me cry on her shoulder.

I felt none of that kind of desperate apprehension on the transplant day though, and I am so grateful. I truly believe the peace I felt made way for prayer, which made way for the news that we got a few hours later.

In the late afternoon, one of the physicians finally came out. He was in blue scrubs, just like you would expect from every TV show or movie you've ever watched. And just like they do in TV shows and the movies, as soon as he announced our name, we all gravitated toward him, like moths to a flame—hoping it was a flame that would not burn us up but would light us instead.

And it did!

"Everything went well," he said. "She's doing well, and you can go in to see her."

The wave of complete relief that washed over me is hard to explain. If I close my eyes and think about that moment, I can still remember it in the fibers of my body—months of despair, stress, and anxiety just flowing out of my body to make way for a new start.

With tears in our eyes, we all went to see Madison. She was just waking up as we got there and was so groggy. And she was still hooked up to IV cords and breathing tubes. The incision was huge; on her tiny body, it was so out of proportion, stretching in the shape of a V from one side of her body to the other. There would be time to worry about that, to take care of it, to help her get through the shock of the sight of it. Right now, I was just so grateful she was alive. I thanked God she was still with us, but I couldn't completely forget that this journey was far, far from over. I couldn't dwell on that though. I had to find some peace and rest in where we were right then. It wasn't easy, but it was needed. Eric was there with us, so it was a moment to find the calm, to harness it and be held inside it.

The truth is that we all need small victories along the way; we need moments where we can breathe and let our guards down and be thankful for what God has given us in the moment.

That's how we feed ourselves; that's how we strengthen ourselves. Even if—or especially if—we know it's the battle that's won, not the war, we must prepare ourselves for the unknowns waiting around the next corner.

Chapter Six

PUTTING ON
THE BOXING GLOVES

L ooking back, I realize that no one promised me smooth
sailing after a transplant, but somehow, I had convinced
myself that it would be. Whether that self-delusion of a
finish line was a coping mechanism or just the fact that I couldn't
mentally project too far forward because it took everything I
had just to get through each day, the result was my holding on to
this dream that once Madison had a new liver, she would have
a new start.

If only all dreams could come true. It wasn't even twenty-
four hours before I realized how wrong I had been. In passing, I
heard one of the doctors speaking about Madison's recovery steps
when he referenced her upcoming chemotherapy appointments.

She had been in chemotherapy since her diagnosis, and
the treatment had taken everything out of her. Every time I had
to bring her into those rooms, sit her three-year-old body in the
oversized recliners, and watch them hook her up to the drip, I felt

devastatingly guilty—here I was, walking her into something we knew was going to deplete her of energy and make her feel sick.

I am so glad I didn't know then, at the outset of treatment, what I know now—of how hard it would be on my heart and soul as a mother. I'm glad I didn't know the extent of how bad it would get watching her go through the treatments. For anyone who has been through chemo or had a loved one go through the process, I know I am speaking to the choir. And then there is always the guilt—even now, reliving these things my daughter had to go through that I couldn't help her with or save her from is so difficult. As she was going through the treatments, there was never an appointment when I didn't sit there hoping and praying that somehow, she would someday understand that we all put her through this with her best intentions at heart.

Naively, I'd assumed the chemotherapy would be finished as soon as the old liver was out. After all, we were so blessed the cancer had not spread to other organs. When the only cancerous organ was removed, it made sense to me that chemotherapy—the treatment to kill cancer cells—could stop.

When I communicated this to one of the doctors, she shook her head no. She was as compassionate as I believe she could be, but it wasn't very much.

After having dealt with so many doctors over the course of Madison's treatment, I feel less offended now by the seeming lack of compassion because I see similarities between all of them. In those similarities, I've come to empathize more with them, and I somewhat understand what their paths have been and how they got to this place where they don't feel.

I want to offer this aside: I say the doctors got to a place "where they don't feel." I'm sure as human beings, they have feelings. That's not what I'm saying. But in the huge impersonal machine of a hospital system, the doctors and residents just become mere cogs in the wheel, there to get a job done and to keep the organization going. I want to believe we had doctors there who cared. The emotionless, impersonal nature of those who worked with us made me feel so ignored, so lost and confused.

From my experience, I've come to see medical school as a sort of fraternity where students are taught to stay within the box of boundaries laid out for them. I've wondered if all that "hazing" separates them too much from the normal people they will someday help, stripping them of their human ability to feel compassion and put themselves in the shoes of the people suffering right in front of them. My daily view was of people who simply didn't have the capacity to care anymore. I would watch their faces, unemotional and distant—what felt, to me, very unhuman.

I couldn't help but wonder what might have been if they could push it all aside and set a goal to truly see the patients, feel empathy for their pain. Would they be able to see or feel their pain and perhaps help them in a completely different way? But that's not the current system. The system we are in hardens doctors from day one, with schools that train the emotion and compassion out of them.

During our time in the hospital, many of the nurses had a glimmer of this true compassion left, but they were dropping like flies—resigning or moving to other departments or other facilities. Every time one who had been kind to us left, my instincts would kick in: How am I going to get my daughter out of here and not let this system destroy or kill us? Failure wasn't an option.

> How am I going to get my daughter out of here and not let this system destroy or kill us?

I felt such an intense resistance and anxiety toward the people helping us. I always felt like the good ones were leaving, and the staff we were then surrounded by just didn't seem to care at all about us in any meaningful way. If my emotions were at an 11, how would I possibly move forward?

I took so much comfort in my research, thinking that it would somehow get all of us to a new place so we could come up with solutions that would keep us from having to repeat the past. Every day I worked those research muscles; I often thought of it in a similar way to working out. I was building strength and preparing us. If I kept getting stronger, then, at some point, I could move us forward.

Even when the mental and physical exhaustion threatened to take me down, I would force myself to snap out of that mentality immediately. There was no way I was giving up—even when the worst-case scenarios showed up at our door.

"She'll have to continue with the chemotherapy, Amy," the doctor explained to me that day. "It's going to be six full rounds." For a moment I sat in confusion, working through mental rebuttals. I ultimately decided against offering them.

Already I had asked for clinical data that the chemotherapy they recommended would help Madison, and even though I asked repeatedly, I was given nothing. That was one of many red flags that began to enter my mind, telling me something wasn't right.

Because I am good at paying attention, I saw these and other discrepancies. The nurses noticed them too. I could tell. But they had about as much ability to speak up in these situations as I did. We all had to pick our battles. When I look back on it now, I see how life was showing me the information I needed at the rate I needed it delivered.

I felt so confused because there was no discussion. The doctor simply stood in our doorway and said that my daughter would die without six full rounds of chemotherapy.

I am a reasonable person, I like to think. But being dismissed without a second thought and then expected to go away was something I didn't feel reasonable about *at all*.

My family members didn't understand this, but I wasn't pushing against *everything* the doctors said to us. When the doctor was telling me that Madison needed six rounds of chemotherapy or she would die and that it would be dangerous to cut this step out, I heard her; I understood what she was saying. I wasn't going to fight them, at that moment, about anything that they said could help Madison's health. But even as I stood there, knowing I would have to go along with what they said, I had that deep gut feeling that this was wrong. My intuition was giving me all the signs, but I didn't go with it.

I was, however, going to keep up my fight for all the details I felt like were getting missed. With her little body just having survived the major transplant surgery, still plugged up to all the machines and with the incision so fresh, I could very clearly see that my energy and resources needed to be steered toward her and her recuperation.

The night after the transplant, I had stayed in her room with her. Zac very much wanted to see her after the surgery was done, but Eric and I agreed she needed to be stable for a period of time before she could get more visitors.

We also weren't sure how Zac was going to handle seeing Madison post-surgery. Since she went into the hospital, he had struggled with the fact that she couldn't leave the hospital. He was definitely old enough to understand that she was sick. But the reality of it was hard for him to stomach. Like all of us, he wanted life to go back to how it was before her diagnosis. He loved being her big brother, but now he never got to see her. And we didn't have any of the answers he wanted to his many questions:

How long until Madison can come home?

When will she be well?

Are you sure she's going to be okay?

The last thing you want to tell your child is that you are asking the same questions he is. That's not the certainty he's looking for.

Once Madison had been stable for a full day, Eric brought Zac up to the hospital. Heartbreakingly, our concerns had been well-founded: The sight of the V incision across her chest and stomach was deeply disturbing for him. I'll never forget how he waited to make sure Madison wasn't looking at him then turned to me with his eyes as wide as saucers. He didn't even think to ask questions—the fear was written all over his face.

Should we have prepared him differently for the sight of it all? Looking back, maybe. It is all hindsight though. In that moment, Eric and I were trying to do our best, but there's no way to know exactly what anyone's feelings or what their reactions will be as life is proceeding. If in everyday life with your child, you don't know exactly what's sticking with them the most, think of this as amplified by what feels like a million. There were so many conversations, sights, questions, and curiosities that could have been weighing on Zac. Eric was with him so much more than I was, but we both really tried to help him know we were there for him.

We also really wanted him to be able to have some space to live too, and not have the weight of his parents constantly asking him if he was okay. To be perfectly honest, if there were moments when he could live without the life and death concerns of his sister, we wanted him to have at least a little taste of that freedom.

Zac loved Madison so much, I'm not sure he ever really stepped away from his worry for her though. He was in school and seeing friends; Eric was doing his best to keep Zac involved in activities and "normal" things for boys his age. Like us, Zac was going through the motions. I didn't realize how much his mind was really on his sister until a few months after Madison's transplant. I was going through his backpack, opening folders that held his work, and I found a picture of Madison in one of his folders. It was taken right after she turned three, at the school she and Zac attended, on a "circus fun day," when they had games, cotton candy, and face painting. Madison had a smile from ear to ear; it took over her whole face and was a truly Madison-sized smile.

When the time was right, I told Zac I found the picture and asked what made him decide to put it in his folder that day.

He remembered the day of the photo like it was yesterday, which revealed the love and determination that Zac still shows as such a loving and caring big brother!

"I don't know, I just wanted to carry it with me," he said.

Sometimes even adults don't know why we do certain things, so for my seven-year-old son, he just needed to see a

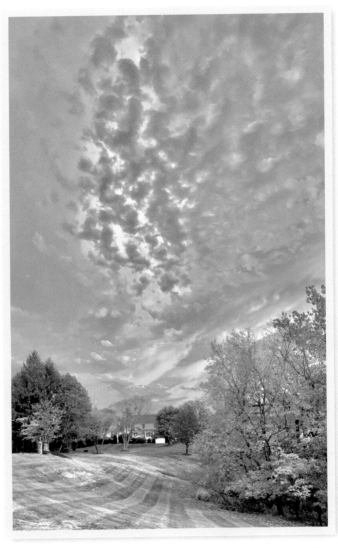

Our son, Zachery, took this from his bedroom window after a storm. It's the perfect representation of our journey.

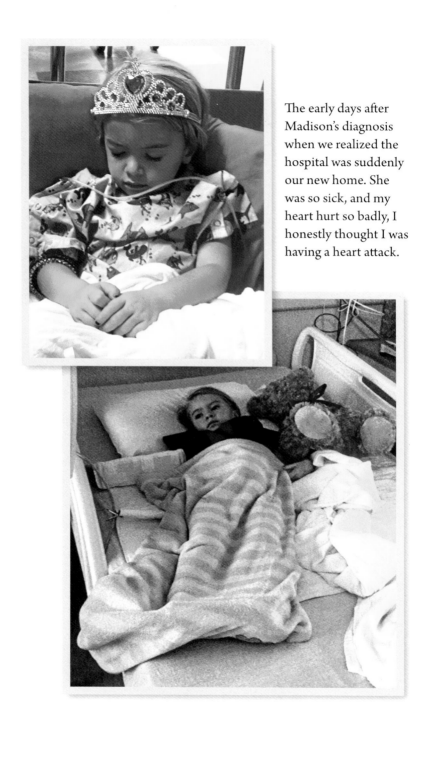

The early days after Madison's diagnosis when we realized the hospital was suddenly our new home. She was so sick, and my heart hurt so badly, I honestly thought I was having a heart attack.

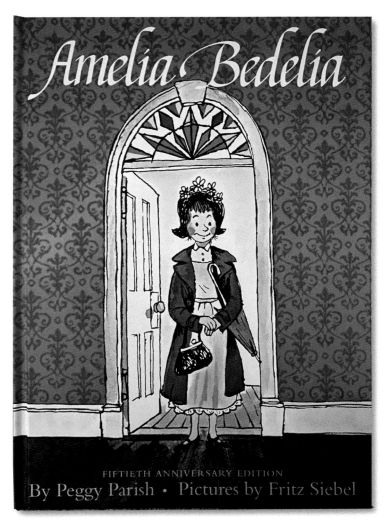

Amelia Bedelia

FIFTIETH ANNIVERSARY EDITION
By Peggy Parish · Pictures by Fritz Siebel

Madison couldn't get enough of books while she was in the hospital. Amelia Bedelia was one of her favorites.

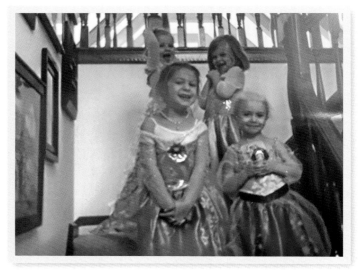

Madison's fourth birthday, only two months after her diagnosis. God gave us an incredible gift of being able to bring her home to celebrate with her friends!

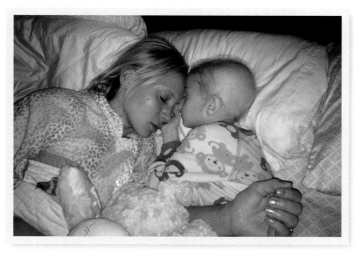

Madison and me. I didn't know that my husband had taken this picture until he showed it to me while we were gathering photos for this book—nine years later.

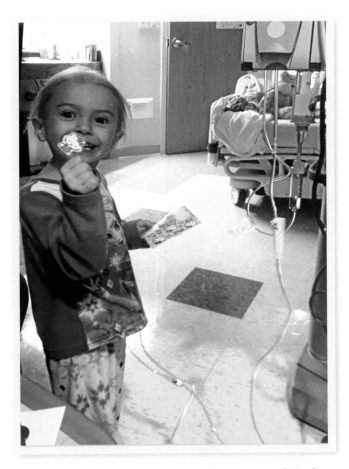

The night before the liver transplant. Eric and Zachery brought dinner to the hospital, and we ate as a family. Madison's courage and her beaming smile gave all of us hope!

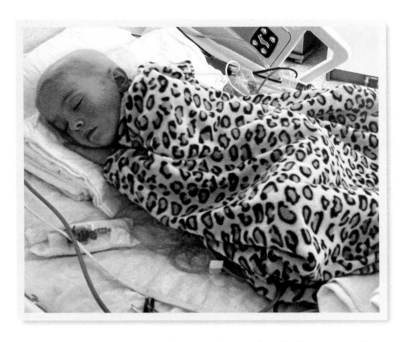

ABOVE: Getting some much-needed rest after the liver transplant. I would watch her sleep, and her peacefulness would wash over me and help me feel calm.

OPPOSITE PAGE: After several days, Madison took a turn and ended up in the Pediatric Intensive Care Unit (PICU), where she was given morphine twice, a drug she's highly allergic to.

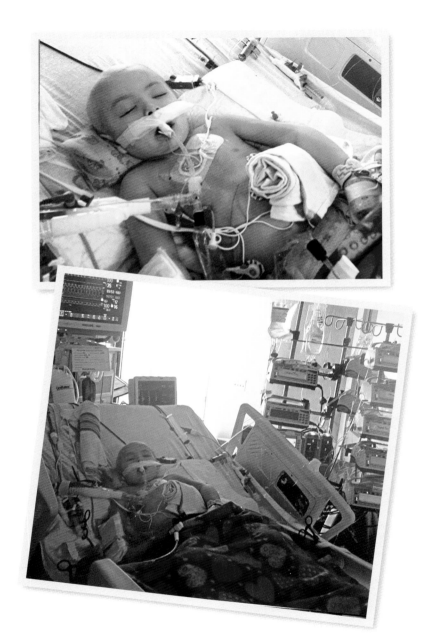

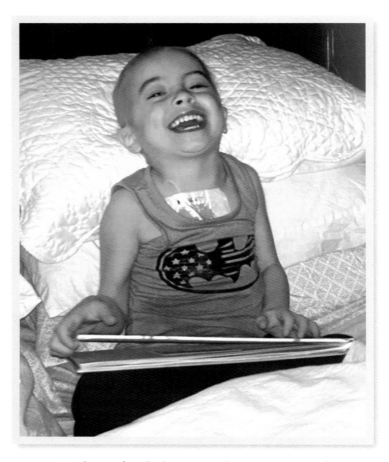

ABOVE: Madison after the liver transplant—we were so happy to see her beautiful smile again!

OPPOSITE PAGE TOP: We were truly blessed to have a day out of the hospital, so we didn't waste it. We took Madison out for a day of fun! Her smile was infectious and gave me courage to know we were going to beat this.

OPPOSITE PAGE BOTTOM: Another fun Day with the family, this time after Madison was released from the hospital.

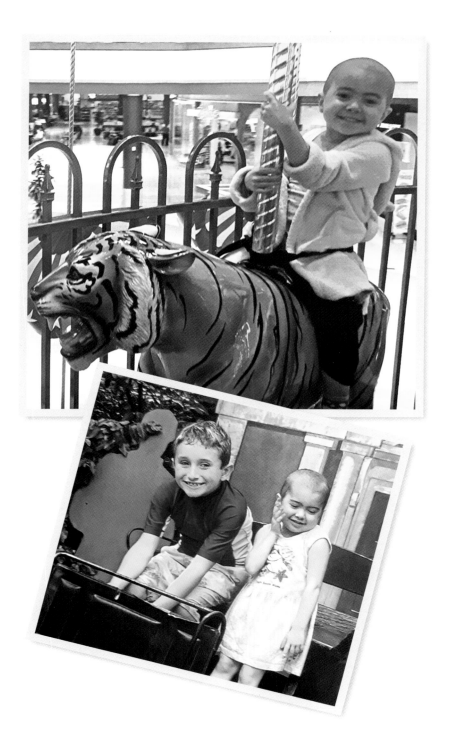

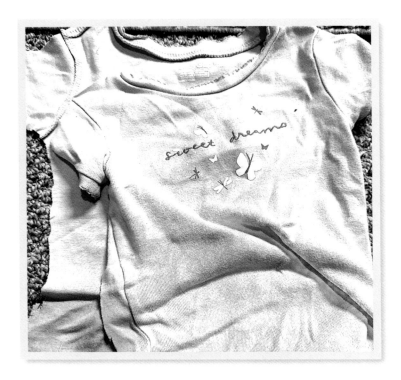

ABOVE: Madison's new shirt was cut off of her after a routine procedure that ended up with her being rushed to the hospital in an ambulance and prepped for surgery.

OPPOSITE PAGE TOP: Madison after six rounds of chemotherapy, declaring, "You can't stop me." After three rounds, she was 19 lbs., her body was frail and thin, and her skin color was off. But she pushed and persevered and completed her six rounds. She's a true superhero!

OPPOSITE PAGE BOTTOM: Madison's chemotherapy completion certificate. She rang the bell on April 17, 2015.

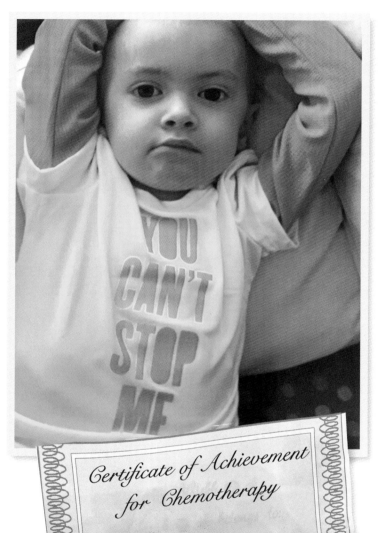

The Make-A-Wish celebration included lunch and a shopping day for Madison and her friends. Unfortunately, the next day's trip to Walt Disney World was canceled (or postponed) when Madison woke up with a 103-degree fever.

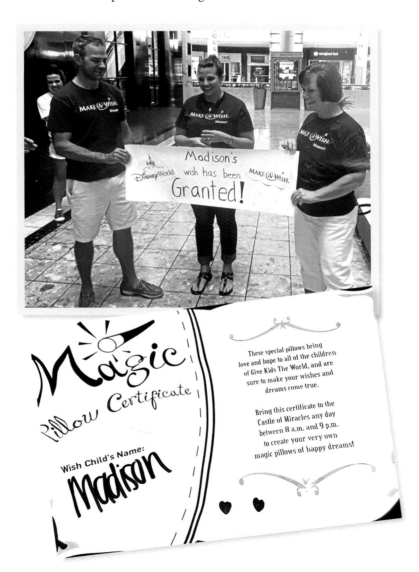

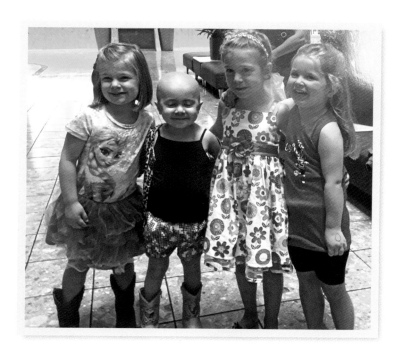

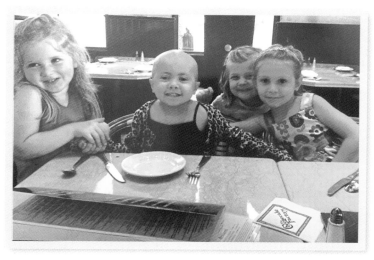

Letters and cards Madison received from her friends at Carmelite and other family friends. Madison and I were greeted with stacks of these each time we were able to come home from the hospital. It meant so much to us.

Dear Madison

We think about you and pray for you every day.

You are very ~~tuff~~ tough and I know that you can get through this ~~tuff~~ tough time. We all believe in you!!! Hope you get better soon!!!

LOVE,
Julia

Dear Madison,
The Carmelite Sisters at your daycare want you to know that they are praying for you. It is not easy to be in the hospital, so we are praying you will feel God's love for you and have peace in His love - felt through your mom & dad. Hope to see you back soon!
In the heart of Jesus
Sr Mary Fresh, SM Guadalupe & other Sisters

GOD HOLDS US IN THE [OF HIS HANDS]

Sept 2014

Dear Madison
Just want you
to know
that I'm thinking
about you.

Please
Get Well Soon

We say a prayer for you every day. We love you very much.
Great GMa + Gpa
Fetsinger
Chris

Warm little wishes
for feeling-better days.

Get Well Soon

See you soon, Madison. We love you
Love,
Grandma + Grandpa

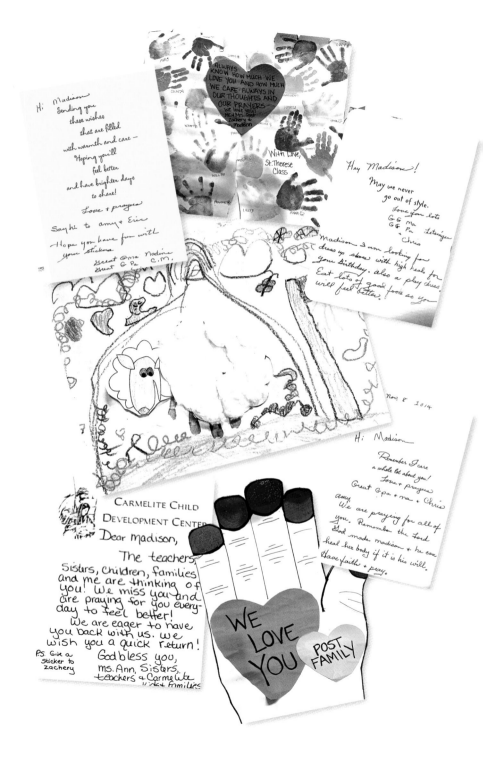

Hi Madison
Sending you
these wishes
that are filled
with warmth and care —
Hoping you'll
feel better
and have brighter days
to share!
Love + prayers
Say hi to amy + Erin
Hope you have fun with
your stickers
Great Gma Nadine
Great G Pa C.M.

ALWAYS
KNOW HOW MUCH WE
LOVE YOU AND HOW MUCH
WE CARE—ALWAYS IN
OUR THOUGHTS AND
OUR PRAYERS—
We love you,
Nick, Mrs. Post,
Zachery +
Madison

With Love,
St. Therese
Class

Hey Madison!
May we never
go out of style.
Love you lots
GG Ma
GG Pa Letanger
+ Chris

Madison I am looking for
dress up shoes with high heels for
your Birthday. also a play dress.
Eat lots of good food as you
will feel better.

Nov. 8 2014

Hi Madison

Remember I care
a whole lot about you!
Love + prayers
Great G pa + ma + Chris
amy.
We are praying for all of
you. Remember the Lord
God made madison + he can
heal her body if it is his will.
Have faith + pray.

CARMELITE CHILD
DEVELOPMENT CENTER

Dear madison,
The teachers,
Sisters, children, families
and me are thinking of
you! We miss you and
are praying for you everyday to feel better!
We are eager to have
you back with us. We
wish you a quick return!

P.S. Give a
sticker to
zachery

God bless you,
Ms. Ann, Sisters,
teachers + Carmelite
Kids + families

WE
LOVE
YOU
POST
FAMILY

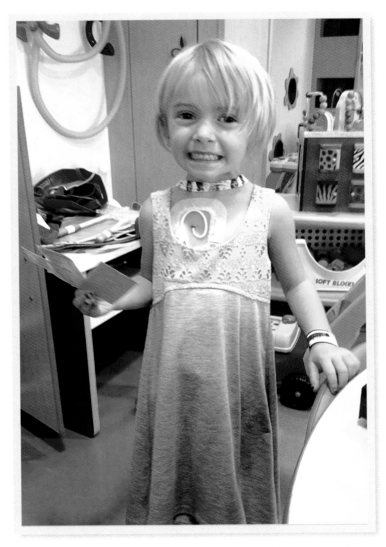

Madison in the hospital's play room. Much of the time Madison was quarantined to her hospital room, but occasionally she was allowed to visit the rooftop garden or to play in the play room.

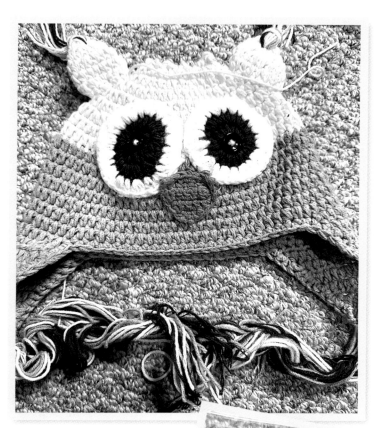

ABOVE: The crocheted owl hat made by a friend. Madison wore it almost every day for a year and a half. It always made her smile.

RIGHT: Nine years later, I found the hospital bracelets I had saved, along with locks of Madison's hair that I had collected as it fell out.

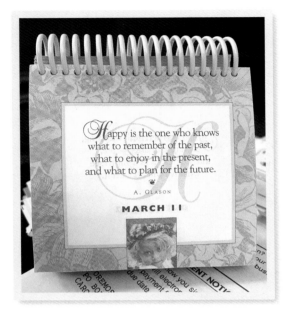

The desk calendar my grandmother gave me when I was in my teens. I carry it everywhere. It gave me great peace during those long dark months and through the years that have followed.

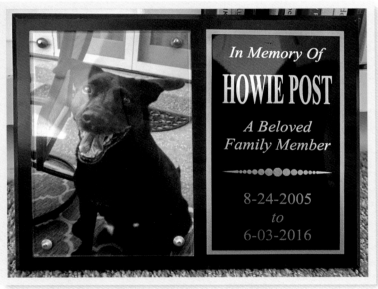

Howie. Eric and I rescued him in 2004, and he became Madison's best friend. The month that Madison rang the bell, Howie was diagnosed with cancer. We lost him two months later, and we were heartbroken. I like to think that he gave up his life in place of Madison.

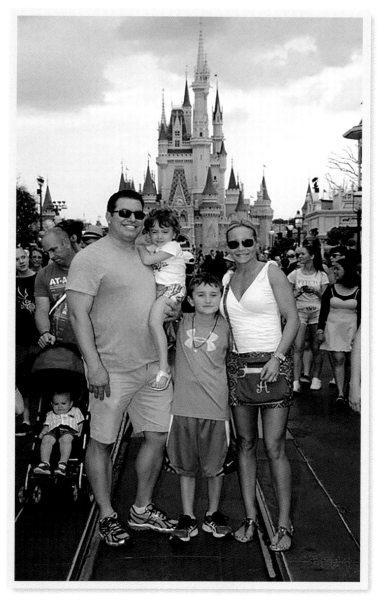

Finally! After several challenging years, Madison was finally able
to have her Make-A-Wish trip to Walt Disney World.

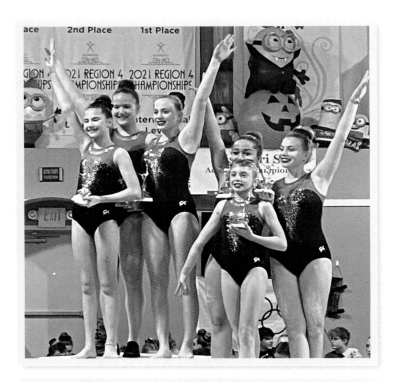

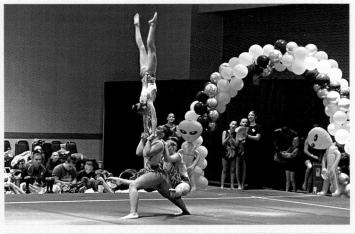

Madison, age twelve, with her acro gymnastics team. By this time, she had been competing for about two years. Madison and her team train all year round for these championship meets. The girls have welcomed Madison and encouraged her to reach for the stars!

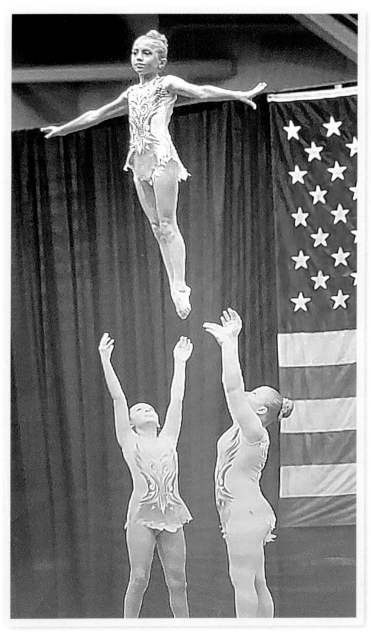

Madison looks like a beautiful angel, able to spread her wings and fly!

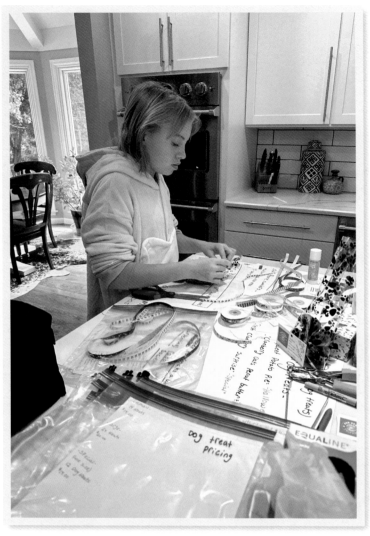

Furr-Ever Friends. Madison making organic dog treats in our kitchen. At thirteen years old, Madison took her pet sitting business to the next level and began to make and sell healthy dog treats. I cherish the time we get to spend togeher in this new business venture, along with the possibilities!

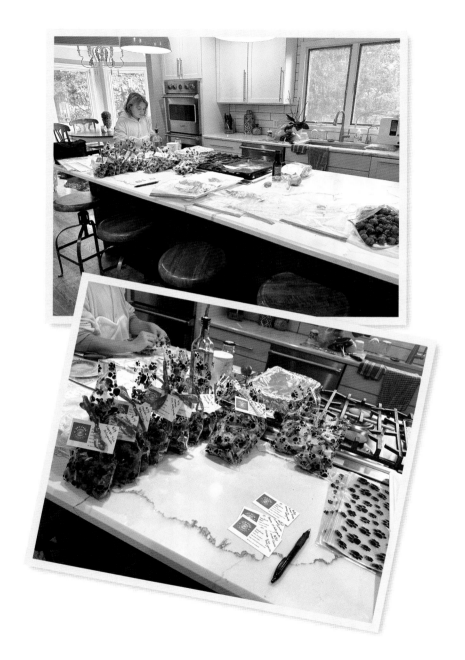

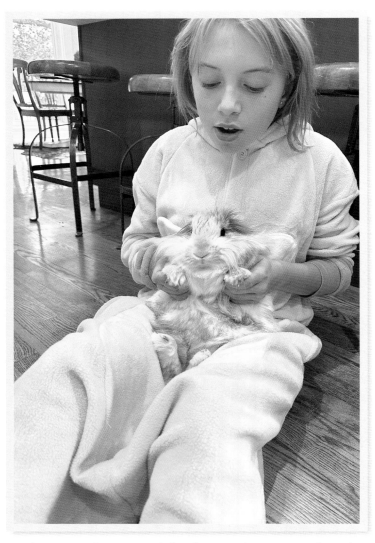

Madison, age thirteen, with her bunny, Thumper. Madison has shown an incredible love for animals and talks about becoming a veterinarian or opening an animal shelter.

picture of Madison smiling, something that reminded him of happier times, not in a hospital room with no ability to leave and no accurate timeframe for when their lives would be normal again.

I definitely had moments when I felt torn in a thousand directions after Eric and Zac would come for dinner and then leave afterward. I wanted Madison and me to be able to leave with them, to get back to our lives. I would feel complete and utter loneliness—mixed with anger, sadness, and despair when they left. We were alone, and I was left to fight this battle. Many times, I couldn't figure out which emotion to feel. What I did know was that I had to hold it together, and there was no time to doddle around. I had work to do to get us out of here. But then moments like those dinner times would remind me that no one was getting back to their lives; all of us were carrying this. We were all having to fight. I might have been the one in the hospital with Madison, but all of us were in a world of complete confusion and sadness. And we were all sleep deprived, which just added to the heaviness. It wasn't the life any of us had expected to live, but we were there, and that's what it was.

I never was much for the saying, "When it rains, it pours," but another round of thunderstorm was heading my way. I was about to have a whole new problem to keep me up at night.

We stayed with the chemo as the doctors had told us to. But as the weeks were moving along, and the realization was hitting me that this wasn't even close to being over, I had to work really hard to find something every day to be grateful for.

Some days when we were reading books or watching movies, it felt like Madison could forget where we were for a bit. But only for a bit.

The transplant happened in October, so in the weeks following it, the ice-skating rink, visible from her room, opened up. We were able to watch people skate, which Madison loved. But it also brought great sadness and even envy the longer we watched them. She wanted to be one of them.

How could I blame her? I felt the same.

I know envy never helps a situation. Our circumstances were just that—ours. And we weren't the skaters out there having fun and living life; we were in the hospital, and we had to try and find ways to be positive there.

What I didn't realize then was that resentment was indeed boiling up within me. It would eventually find a place to settle and would stay for many years. I didn't know how to recognize it, much less cope with it. I had no concept of how much damage could be done by not recognizing it.

But when would I find time to address what I was going through? I didn't have time to sleep, let alone deal with my feelings. All that time, when I thought I was just pushing it away, God was working in me. He knew I needed to address these things, but

He also knew how stubborn I was and how determined I was to focus on my daughter. I feared that if I took my eyes off Madison for even a second, I would fail her.

> *All that time, when I thought*
> *I was just pushing it away,*
> *God was working in me.*

That's the thing about me—I have a long history of feeling like I am failing even when I am succeeding. We all have our hangups; I certainly had many that would creep up and hold on longer than I wanted. To this point, my job had just barely been hanging on. As I mentioned, my clients were so gracious in staying with me. Every time I contacted them, I would ask them to please not give up on me, and I would promise that I would be back to 100 percent soon. Not only would they reply with promises to wait, but they would also ask me how I was doing.

Talk about things to be grateful for!

I was holding on to that promise I was making to my clients—and myself: Yes, I *would* be back to 100 percent. And soon.

At that point, I'd been selling aesthetics products for over a decade. And even though I had switched companies a couple times, my clients—or the people I sold to—followed me. So these people had been with me, some of them for years. They knew me. They understood that what I was living through was really difficult and that I asked for something many may not—I humbly asked for my clients not to give up on me, to believe in me, because they had known me for many years, and we were not only business partners, but we were friends.

Part of being in the hospital with Madison meant I wasn't really up on behind-the-scenes happenings at my company. I wasn't ever a huge one on company gossip, but I had my friends at work, and of course, I usually liked to keep tabs on what was going on. That was an easy thing to let go of when my attention needed to shift to Madison.

So I had heard murmurings about some problems in the company. Patent issues aren't completely abnormal in that line of work, so I let it go in one ear and out the other. What I didn't realize was that what had started with some patent issues would result in my company being unable to sell a particularly well-regarded product for a whole year! Not only could they not sell it, but for that year, we, the salespeople, wouldn't be able to talk about it either.

I'm giving a super top-level overview here just to help you understand what was going on. Imagine how you would feel if you've been buying a product regularly from the same company. Then suddenly you can't buy it, and your trusted salesperson can't even talk about it. To put it mildly, clients were put out. And the people in management were trying to figure out ways to deal with the significant amount of money that was being hemorrhaged as a result.

Mind you, I was hearing of all this, but it wasn't really worrying me because I had so many other things worrying me. It's like "take a number," and this particular number was not anywhere near ready to be served.

But then one day, while Madison and I were on a twenty-four-hour release (why these little pockets of time at home always seemed to be plagued by an exterior problem, I'll never understand) that number got called.

It was that evening, and since we were going back to the hospital the next day, I was doing my best to get some things done. I can still see it—I was walking across my bedroom with my phone in my hand, and I opened up my email just to give it a quick check. I swiped on the email from my company. Thank goodness my bed was right there for me to drop down on; otherwise, when my knees gave out, I surely would have hit the floor.

They were letting me go.

Have you ever been let go from a job? Humiliating. Surprising. World ending. Trust me, being fired by email makes all those bad emotions feel even worse. Especially when I had done such good work for that company for so long. I'd made them great money and brought them the very best clients. There was nothing in my performance that warranted this.

I closed the email, threw my phone on the bed like I couldn't get away from it fast enough. I forced myself to take a deep breath, then I grabbed the phone again and quickly reopened the email.

Had it really said what I thought it did?

One more read confirmed it.

This was more than losing a job. This was the career I had been building, the salary we depended on; it was our family's health insurance.

Thinking about the health insurance made my chest get so tight I could hardly breathe. The letter explicitly stated I would have options for COBRA, but I knew the prices for COBRA would be astronomical compared to what we had been paying.

Then there was the company car! Sure, it had been sitting idle in the garage at the children's hospital most of the time, but I still needed it. A car had always been part of my job, but now, in a flash, it was being taken away. The email gave directions to leave the keys under the mat, and someone would come to my house and get it.

Everything down to the last detail was laid out in that email. It was horrifying, a truly terrifying moment. We were barely holding on, and it was like the last bit of the rug was pulled out from under us.

As soon as I could speak, I yelled for Eric. He must have been able to hear the undertones—well, outright panic—in my voice, because he was there in an instant.

"What's going on?" he asked. "Are you okay?"

I couldn't stomach saying any more bad news out loud. I was crying and shaking at this point. I could barely hand over my phone for him to read the email for himself. All I could say was, "I'm sorry." And I was. I was sorry for this situation. That he was going to have to go through it. That Zac and Madison would have to feel like another layer of security was gone from their lives. For the whole mess. I was so irrevocably sorry. I had failed my family, especially my daughter.

I couldn't stop the crying or the uncontrollable shaking in my hands. I just sat on the bed until the room finally came back into focus.

As soon as Eric understood what was going on, he quickly told me there was nothing for me to be sorry about. We sat in our room for a while, just letting it sink in. We didn't immediately talk about options or what the plan would be, and I was grateful for that—grateful he gave me time to gather myself and find some kind of center instead of giving into emotions and letting them take control.

The company offered a good severance package: one year of salary and health insurance. Once it all sank in, I still didn't know what I was going to do, but I knew my plan would not include signing the deal the company had sent over. I knew if I signed it, I would be agreeing that what they were doing was okay. I'd be signing away my ability to come back to them and say, "Hey, this is wrong."

Believe me, part of me was thinking: Do not turn down the severance package. Take what you can get.

My intuition was the voice I was learning to trust, and I was going to listen to where it guided me. I was angry, heartbroken, and scared to death. As if I could be more scared, considering what we had been going through for the past five months—but our story just kept getting worse. I was flat-out tired of feeling like we were getting the short end of the stick.

Maybe if I was a different person, I could have signed the offer. I could have said, "Something better will come tomorrow." But I have never been that person. I've never backed down from much of anything, so I guess I must have subconsciously decided *Why start now?*

Sometimes I think that our actions are the results of our surrounding circumstances, and in different situations we would react differently. Maybe that's true. I also feel people are all unique in how we react to situations, but there are threads that run throughout. I've found Madison is like me; she doesn't back down. No matter the situation, she's going to keep fighting.

In this set of circumstances I was in, the idea of letting a large company get away with something like this—letting me, and what I imagined was a large number of employees, go in order to make up for poor decision-making on their part was wrong. We weren't numbers. We were people. And with families to support on top of it!

As soon as I told Eric of my decision, I braced myself. It seemed over the last months that we hadn't agreed on when I should be speaking up and advocating and when I should stay quiet. To my surprise, there was no disagreement on this. We were on the same page. We would fight this legally.

"It's going to be hard to find a lawyer who wants to go up against pharma," I said.

I knew in my heart this was going to be challenging, but I hadn't completely given up on the world of underdogs. They were out there; surely the lawyering world had a few to be found in it as well.

I had heard about one guy in New York who was willing to take on pharma companies, but that felt like a long shot. There was also one guy—just one!—locally who people said might take the case. I reached out to him, sent him all the information, and after a day I got his answer: he would try it.

I wish I could say I felt like this was a victory, but I knew what we were signing up for. There was no celebration. This could be very good or very bad, depending on how I played my cards. My thoughts were like a tornado in my head. Could I actually do this with everything that was taking place with Madison? Could I effectively participate in this case and still stay focused on her? I'm not sure I was even capable of thinking straight due to sleep deprivation. And if I couldn't think straight, was it really the time for a lawsuit against a huge pharma company? Was I nuts? Perhaps. But I wasn't someone to be pushed around or messed with. I'd seen it time and again in the hospital with Madison—mothers with sick children have incredible strength, strength perhaps they wouldn't have known they had until they had to use it. When I thought and prayed about it, I knew: this was my time.

Immediately my lawyer and I were talking on a daily basis. I was trying to paint the picture for him and give him absolutely all the information I had. Technically, I'd been on medical leave when the firing happened, but even with this key fact, the lawyer said there wasn't much of a case. In the state of Missouri, you can fire anyone for any reason. I took that contract the company had sent over, ripped it into shreds, and threw it in the trash.

> *I'd seen it time and again in the hospital*
> *with Madison—mothers with sick children*
> *have incredible strength, strength perhaps*
> *they wouldn't have known they had*
> *until they had to use it.*

I knew I had to fight like hell to get through this. I questioned how I would keep this from destroying me. In the last five months, I had already faced so many obstacles, and now this. Familiar feelings of loneliness and terror began coming over me again: Was I going to fail my family? I knew that sometimes, no matter how hard you fight, it's impossible to change the world and make it more fair. Would this turn out positive or negative?

I felt like David up against Goliath, with one little slingshot up against the beast. I don't know what happened exactly, but I remember the moment a positive energy settled over me about the whole case. Was it God coming to rescue me and breathe new life into me, showing His presence? I believe so. With that positive energy I pushed myself forward. From then on, there simply wasn't any more questioning of the details and whether or not it was wise to be taking on this fight. In the end I think that was the best place to be. Sometimes you just don't know what you don't know—you simply have to go for it!

Starting then, all communication with my company had to go through my attorney. I was fine with that. But it did mean he was my lifeline, and the only way I was able to talk to him was from my phone in the hospital. I felt a real loss of control, and even though I am not good with that feeling, I trusted that this was what God had planned. I believed that sense of peace had come over me for a reason. The most common sight in those days was me pacing up and down the hallway outside Madison's room on my cell phone, painstakingly going over the smallest details, just playing back every moment of recent years so we could figure out our case.

All this time on the phone meant I had to leave Madison's room more than usual, which didn't prove to be easy. I felt like I was being pulled in so many directions. Madison's emotions were starting to be more of a roller coaster, which was understandable, given how trapped she felt after months and months of being locked up and having no firm answers on whether it would ever end. Unfortunately, I could never tell when the drops of the roller coaster were coming. My ability to adapt and stay on my toes was crucial, because every day I had to go into the legal fight swinging. Perhaps because I'd already been fighting so hard for Madison for months, it was just my state of mind. It wasn't hard to find that intensity in me.

Early on I remember feeling like my attorney wasn't matching me on my level of aggression and the fight I wanted to give. I vividly remember his soft, kind demeanor at the outset, but I needed him to step that up as the fight went on. Even when I knew very little about him or his personality, I knew enough to tell him one day, "I don't need a kitty cat right now. I need a tiger. You are going to have to be a tiger for me."

I remember the conversation went quiet, but I think he got the message. After I spoke up, he was different, better. I wasn't looking for cutthroat, mind you. But I did want him to be aggressive.

It's funny how when you are just living life and doing what you have to do, sometimes you don't realize the effect you are having on people. A few years ago, my husband and I were at a friend's pool party. We were just getting to know one of the couples there, and the women asked me about Madison being sick. I said something to the effect of, "Yes, in the process I had to get a lawyer for a work situation. It was a truly awful situation, a very hard time."

The man looked at me and asked, "Who was your attorney?"

When I told him the name, he shook his head, laughing at the coincidence. Apparently, my attorney was defending this man's company at the time. The attorney had told the man about my case and then said, "She was the most memorable client I ever had."

I'll give it to that attorney; it was a memorable ending for sure.

After six months of back and forth and stressful, up-all-night worries and digging through the past, the company's attorneys called us to a meeting. We were all sitting at this long table, and even though I was terrified of how it was going to go, I knew I was in the right. I shouldn't have been fired, and I was not going to be bullied by this company just because they were bigger. I'd had it with bullies! I'd had it with systems that wanted to keep hard-working individuals down! I wanted to jump across that table and pounce those smug expressions off their faces, but I kept my composure.

They had an offer. I turned it down.

After the meeting, my attorney kept telling me I didn't have a case and that I should take what they were offering. I guess you could say I had been through enough with the hospital administration that I didn't need to take anything else! I had to pull out the boxing gloves and get creative. I went back to my attorney with one last negotiation.

At that point he didn't know what to make of me, but he took it to the company.

Soon, he came back to me and said the case was settled. "You just won more free money than any of my clients have ever won," he said.

Man, did that comment make me livid! I let him know straightaway that money wasn't free. I worked decades for my career, my clients, and my reputation. What the company did was wrong and needed to be righted. If not for that, *what is our justice system even for*?

Chapter Seven

SURVIVING STORMS

L ife isn't fair.

It's a saying we've all heard before. Some of us would say it's much more than a saying—it's a truth. And I would agree.

What always strikes me about that saying, or truth, is that the only people who wrestle with it are the ones who have struggles. People who wake up every day and have a pretty good life—the kind of people who things come easy for—they probably never have to wrestle with whether life is fair, and then what to do with that. They never have to dig deep to decide if they are going to keep living life and loving life even in the midst of its unfairness.

I think it's easy to stand back and say that's the line that divides people: you are a person who has either struggled and has faced the unfairness of life, or you're not. In my life I've been tempted to think this way, but ultimately, I've decided it's not correct. I think what really defines those of us who have struggled in life is whether we can look at the unfairness of life, at the unfairness of whatever hand has been dealt to us, and not let that make us bitter.

For me, that's the line. If you're standing in the middle of the storm, are you cursing the fact that the hurricane came to your zip code? Or can you stand in the middle of the storm, wind whipping around you, rain drenching you to the bone, all your belongings being flung away, and every one of your plans destroyed, *and still praise God?*

That's the test, and oh, how I wish it was a test we could pass once and be done with. But that doesn't seem to be the way the world works. Instead, we go through the process again and again, and every time we must come back to our center and remind ourselves what life is about, what we value. We must take ourselves by the shoulders (because in the middle of the worst storms we are so often alone and have to give ourselves our own pep talks) and remind ourselves that this is no time to get angry or wrapped up in how we were wronged. Instead, we must look at what's swirling around us, make a plan that helps us and the ones we love, and push forward.

> *We must look at what's swirling around us, make a plan that helps us and the ones we love, and push forward.*

144

The first time I stood in a storm like this was way before Madison was sick. It was before Zac or Madison were born, and even before I knew Eric. It was after I tried to tell my parents that my brother, Chad, was sick with an addiction—when they ignored my attempts to tell them what was going on so we could band together as a family and help him.

That afternoon, and then in the weeks, months, and years after, was the first time I really experienced a storm. Emotionally, I felt a complete upheaval. I was so hurt at how my parents treated me, but also at how I felt they were treating Chad! Didn't they want to help him? Didn't they know me well enough to see I was trying to help him? I knew our family wasn't perfect. What family is? But I had thought at the end of the day, we all would be able to get on the same page in a time of crisis.

These were the feelings of a sixteen-year-old crying out for help. Unfortunately, those feelings of abandonment, being ignored, and feeling inconsequential followed me for many years. I had found myself standing alone in the storm. I felt beaten up daily, confused about how to go on. And it was only during the writing of this book that I have felt a release. I realized that I needed to forgive my parents. I love them very much, and I would never want to hurt them. Through my own experiences, I am reminded every day that nobody is perfect. We all have our challenges. My parents had to deal with the sickness of addiction in their child, while I have had to face cancer in mine.

I am thankful, though, that in the situation with my parents, I did not get bitter to the point of giving up and becoming a victim. Instead, I used what I experienced as a time of strengthening and organizing. I can look back and see that the conversation in the living room was the beginning of a six-year wind-up to leaving home and living on my own, and later building a life that I wanted, where family would value each other and fight for one another when anyone was in need.

It was painful, so painful, to watch what was happening to Chad back then. His attitude changes were getting worse—he was even more withdrawn and more openly rebellious to my parents. Any capacity for a friendship with me was long gone. Our family would get phone calls in the middle of the night, and I'd be the one to answer. I was sixteen or seventeen, and Chad would be begging someone to come get him or to bring him money or, even more common, bail him out of jail. (My parents chose to bail him out for more years than I can remember.) And when one of us did pick him up, his wasn't the kind of situation where you got him home, he slept it off, and he repented and changed his ways the next day. The addiction and drug abuse were fierce. His spiral was downward, and everyone except my parents could see it—or rather, they didn't *want* to see it.

Chad's first child was born when he was only sixteen. I give the mother of that child credit, though. She was the only person in Chad's life who didn't let him get away with his behavior. He didn't want to deal with having a child, but she wasn't going to let that be okay. All she wanted was for him to come meet the baby. She gave him a little time, but he wouldn't do it. Then Chad went to prison. Later, when he got out, she went to court and got him for all the back child support he owed. I wish that would have been a wake-up call for him.

Prison. A child he doesn't know. If it had been a wake-up call for my parents, at least, maybe something could have changed. But everyone just kept throwing money at Chad, asking him to use it for getting his life together. Of course, he didn't. He used it to keep his addiction alive.

Anytime I tried to bring up helping Chad, I would get the same response—it was denial at this point and would be for many years. And this is after he had gone to prison many times! After we had watched him spend years locked up. Yet the patterns weren't changing.

Chad went on to have children with three other women. He didn't have much of a hand in raising any of them. Drugs and prison seemed to be his choices and patterns. Dalton was Chad's second child, and he changed things in my family. Dalton's mother was as sick as Chad, so they both lost custody of Dalton; they weren't fit to raise a child. My mom wanted custody, and I understood why: Dalton was so, so sick. He would spend every other weekend with us, and every time we had him, he would be sick and need medical attention due to the neglect by his parents. He had ear infections. He had stomachaches. And he had crying fits because something—everything—hurt.

When my mother formally asked for custody from the state, I asked her if she knew what she was doing. The storm was all around us all the time, and if she wasn't willing to try and help her son, who was causing it—to even speak the truth about what was happening—I couldn't help but wonder what was going to happen if she had Chad's child in the house.

My mother was not willing to discuss it. "This is what's happening; don't ask about it."

Conversation closed; don't return to it. I'd been down that road with her before, and I knew she was serious, so I held my tongue and stepped back.

That was the beginning of the heartrending end for our family. We had all been living in a state of toxic silence, but once Dalton got involved, the contradictions and blatant denials were so obvious. It just ate away at all of our relationships. The drugs physically destroyed Chad, but the effects of his addiction destroyed the rest of us.

Eventually I learned to live within this storm. Like I said, I wasn't bitter, but there was definitely a lot of hurt and pain to walk through. My brother was the favorite. His life was a mess, and the entire family would do anything to help. I was working my tail off in school and trying to build a life for myself. When I was fifteen, I started a lawn mowing business because I knew I was going to need money. Then when my parents stopped paying attention to me because of the Chad situation, I threw myself into work even more. Some part of me knew that working, making money, and being independent was going to be the only way I could get out. So I put everything I had toward that end.

It would have been so easy for me to go the way Chad went. I could have been like, "Oh, well, if my parents aren't going to pay attention to me for doing the right things, I'll do the wrong things and see if I can start getting some of their love."

That kind of decision is what plenty of people make—people who are just like me. Same upbringing. Same opportunities or lack of them. Why does one go left and one go right? Plenty of people have theories, but I think it boils down to what we can't actually know—it's something with God, something in how we are made, something we ourselves can't take credit for. I will say I am so grateful for it though. To this day, I thank God for it.

Toward the end of high school, I was working for a tanning salon in town. Around the time I graduated, the tanning salon went up for sale. I was hoping to go to college, but I knew it wasn't going to happen straightaway. My parents and grandparents were always offering to pay for Chad's college, or they were buying him vehicles so he could get back and forth to a job. Those offers weren't there for me.

Immediately I saw how the tanning salon could help—I'd been working there long enough that I had seen all the ways it could become more profitable. I'd never had formal business training, but I'd been doing research in my own way. Observing, listening, watching. I saw where the gaps were, and I knew I could work hard enough to fix them. If I started making a profit,

I could pay for school, and I could save money to move to a bigger city.

I went to my parents to ask for a loan so I could purchase the business, but before the words were out of my mouth my mother said no.

"What do you know about owning a business?" she asked.

I hadn't done it before—she was right—but I knew a lot about working. I knew about showing up for shifts when you didn't want to. I knew about taking out a loan from the bank for a car because no one would help you. I knew about standing in a storm and making a way out for yourself. I knew about moving forward instead of getting buried in bitterness. There was no changing her mind though.

Luckily my dad felt differently. He thought about my request for a while and then agreed to the loan. As soon as my mom caught wind of it, she set up a steep amortization, telling me it had to be paid back in five years. Here was that decision again: Would I get consumed with the unfairness of the situation, or would I spend that energy moving forward? I went forward and was able to pay back their loan in four.

All in all, I owned the salon for six and a half years, and I somehow managed to do eighteen hours a semester in college as well. The whole time, I was working hard at the salon and in school, but I was also working hard to get past the hurt of what had happened in our home. All my extra time went to helping my mom with Dalton. He spent most days with me at the tanning salon. Then on the weekends, we would spend time riding bikes, playing, or whatever he wanted to do. His road was hard from the start. Having been born to a mother who was a drug addict had resulted in health problems he could never quite shake. As he got older, he had anger at having been abandoned by both parents. But even when he was a child, I could see the bitterness taking hold.

I loved my nephew more than anything in the world—he was my little buddy and companion. But when the time came for me to get out of the small town and leave for St. Louis, I knew I had to give myself a shot at the life I wanted. I had sold the salon and had money that could get me started in St. Louis. My classes would transfer to college there as well.

Everything was lining up, and I could see that it was everything I had been working for. In many ways, it was everything I had wanted to prove since that day in our living room when I tried to tell my parents Chad was in trouble. I was able to build a life. I was able to start with nothing and end up a woman with a successful business she had sold at a great profit.

Life hadn't started out fair, but I wasn't bitter or angry. Unfairness had been an advantage because I never expected to stay where I was. There is a respect and meaning that comes with working hard and not being handed everything without having put in the effort. My brother was doomed from the start by all the handouts, money, vehicles, clothes, everything being thrown at him with a hope that he would get his life together. How was being an enabler ever going to help my brother or our family? This truly frustrated me and broke my heart. It would eventually be a topic that would haunt my mother and father for decades. Maybe my parents begged God for that "handbook" the same way I did years later with my own child. They didn't receive it. But the thing is, these situations don't get better if you stick your head in the sand or brush things under the rug waiting for the quick fix. They tear families apart. This situation certainly ripped mine apart.

> *Life hadn't started out fair,*
> *but I wasn't bitter or angry.*
> *Unfairness had been an advantage*
> *because I never expected to stay where I was.*

I'd found a way out of that family storm, though, and learned enough that when the next storm came, I'd have experience under my belt. As always, none of that made the hurt of what was happening easier to bear. I remember the day I drove away from my parents' house for good. Dalton was riding his tricycle as fast as he could, following my vehicle to the end of the gravel road. I cried for the whole three-hour drive to my new home in St. Louis.

Chapter Eight

LEARNING TO SPEAK UP

The whole time my case with my former employer was proceeding, the most important events were unfolding inside the hospital with Madison. Even though the case was high stakes for our family, there were no higher stakes than the fight she was undertaking every single day.

She was recovering well from the transplant, but the chemotherapy was taking it out of her. It was wearing her little body down to a point where we found ourselves locked in a vicious cycle. The chemotherapy made her weak, and her immune system was down, so she would pick up any illness going around the hospital. But when there was a break from the chemotherapy, we couldn't really celebrate the break because we were not allowed to leave the hospital over concern that Madison could become even sicker.

That first Christmas was rough. We were ready to go home on Christmas Eve—Madison had her heart set on it, and so did I. We were waiting, bags packed and dressed to leave, when the doctors came in.

"We're sorry, her levels aren't good. We will need you to stay," one of them said.

It was what we heard so much of the time: "Her levels aren't good." Looking back on it now, with what I've learned about how all those medicines were interacting with her body, causing a storm at every turn, it's a miracle her levels were *ever* good! I know they were being cautious, and we wanted that caution to a point. If numbers were scary, then yes, of course, let's do whatever we need to do. But there were times when something was spiking or was a little off, that they still wanted a load of tests. She was taking so many medications, her liver didn't stand a chance of processing all that was flowing through her!

When you're a parent, those "in charge" make it virtually impossible to question what they say. Mind you, that's coming from someone who is a fighter. My heart goes out to any parent who doesn't have that fighting instinct. As soon as they start talking about numbers, there's just no way to combat that information.

> *When you're a parent,
> those "in charge" make it
> virtually impossible
> to question what they say.*

After the doctors left, I had to gather my thoughts for a moment before I could bear to look at Madison. Eric's family was at the house already, waiting for us. And Madison had so excitedly been thinking about being home with her brother, and about opening their presents together on Christmas morning. On top of that, it had snowed. After months of watching ice skaters out the window, she'd had it—she wanted to be playing in that snow!

Sometimes all you can do is hug your child because any positive thing you say would be a lie. I was not going to give Madison untruths. I needed her to know I was someone she could always rely on, a voice she could always trust. So I hugged her; I told her we were going to have a special Christmas (which wasn't a lie), and then when I felt like she was feeling at least a little better, I left the room to call Eric and tell him the news.

One of the nurses told me I could go downstairs to a room that was set up with gifts for the kids. She stayed in the room while Madison slept so I could go downstairs and explore the options. There was table after table of gifts—toys, clothes, princess dresses, any sports-related gift you can think of—everything a kid could ever want. All the gifts were great, but I knew none of it was what Madison wanted. She just wanted to be home. The volunteers were so kind. I chose a couple of things I thought Madison might enjoy, and they said they would wrap them and deliver them to the room.

I remember it feeling like an almost out-of-body experience as I returned to Madison's room, thanked the nurse, and watched her leave. I was then left there for the rest of the night while my daughter slept. Was this really our Christmas Eve? Why did it feel like we were trapped here? I was going to have to stay positive and strong, but that was a breaking point. How were we ever going to get out of this hospital?

Our family arrived early the next morning with a big cooler of all kinds of food Eric's company had purchased for us. A "paper plate Christmas" is what we called it, complete with little red Dixie cups. None of us were okay with it, but we all tried to stay positive because, after all, it was Christmas. It wore on Eric's father though. He was visibly struggling; I understood the feeling—the hospital is a scary place to be, even scarier when your granddaughter is in the middle of a gutting round of chemotherapy and looking withered and weak, stuck in a hospital bed.

After they left, I remember having a complete and total feeling of being trapped. It was the first time I had felt it that intensely. That anger at our situation was raw and very real. I can't speak for Madison and how she felt, but my mother's intuition saw some of the same feelings in her. That Christmas night, she was a different sort of quiet. Try as I might to speak to her and reach into the part of her that was shutting down, there wasn't a thing I could say. We watched the snow and sat with our gifts and ate leftovers from the cooler.

And after she fell asleep, I whispered, like always, "I love you." It was the truth times a million.

Of course, in a hospital, time stops for nothing. They decorate as best they can and give the kids gifts, but the day after Christmas, everything is back to normal. It could be a Tuesday in October or a Saturday in June. It was just another hospital day.

In my gut, I felt like something about the hospital was making and *keeping* her sick. So many times, we were quarantined in her room to keep her free of illness. We would obey; we would stay there and not leave for any of the things she liked. No visits to the playroom or the rooftop garden. No walking the halls. It was just days upon weeks of coloring books, Disney movies, and watching ice skaters out the window. Madison slept a lot, and I had many hours of silence, time to myself, which was both good and bad.

But then, even after our vigilance in keeping her away from people, she would still catch something. It didn't make sense to me until we were in the middle of another quarantine period. I sat in that room and watched all the nurses and doctors coming in and out. That whole time it had been right under my nose! They were the only ones coming in and out. *They* were the ones bringing in whatever was getting Madison sick!

My daily dialogue with my lawyer really had me stirred up, so my senses were heightened toward injustice in every direction. When I realized how the nurses and doctors might be contributing to Madison's situation, I spoke up. In the same way I had spoken up about the nutrition, I started with asking questions of the nurses I trusted. I wanted to know about precautionary measures they took against bringing germs from one room to the next. Then I asked about past and present protocols as well as the number of kids coming down with the same strands of illnesses. Once I felt like I had a pretty good picture of how things were done and coupled that with research I'd done on my own, I started calling meetings with the hospital administration.

Change wasn't swift, but it did come. At the times that Madison was more vulnerable to illness, doctors and nurses started suiting up in protective gear before they came into our room. It made a difference in her resilience against disease. It also gave me a small boost of confidence—advocating for her was worth it.

Someone who understood and supported me in this effort was Kim. We were still texting every night, and when there was any victory at all, we would relish in it. Both of us knew that in these lives we were living with our sick daughters, every win counted.

The celebration was brief though. There was another threat, and it was very literally knocking on our door.

One evening, a resident physician came into our room at 2:34 a.m. The moment he entered the room, the air changed, and the hair on the back of my neck stood up. I was used to how the residents would enter our room without warning, so I knew I wasn't so much bothered about that. It was something very specific to this person and the feeling he gave off.

Madison was sleeping, and I was sitting still in the chair in the corner of the room. The doctor saw me and didn't say a word. He just lurked around, staring at things and picking them up as though he was looking for something. When he finally did speak, he began asking the most unusual questions.

I was so sleep deprived, and it being the middle of the night, I could barely focus. But his presence made the blood in my veins feel electric, and heightened all my senses.

I asked him what he was looking for because he continued to rifle around. He said he just needed to ask a few more questions. Again, the questions were random and disjointed. None of them helped me make sense of his behavior. When he left, I was out of breath, and my skin felt cold and clammy. And I was *angry*.

The next morning, one of the doctors came into our room, and I told her about the experience. I expressed my concerns and relayed that I was uncomfortable with this person. Something was very wrong, and I trusted my instincts. Over the months we had had hundreds of residents, doctors, and nurses in our room. I had come to understand what the general line of questions were. His, though, had been totally irregular and downright strange.

The doctor asked me what my problem was. She restated that the man was a resident, as though that information in and of itself should be proof enough that there was no problem. Her tone conveyed to me that I was bothering her and challenging her in a way I shouldn't.

I was not going to back down though. I told her about my instinctive feeling, how strange the man acted, and the unusual questions he asked. She told me he would be coming back each evening on his rounds. I knew this was completely unacceptable. I didn't want to be within fifty feet of that guy again, and I sure didn't want him anywhere near my daughter.

I told the doctor very clearly that the resident was not allowed in Madison's room again. And she reiterated that he would be making his rounds again that night; there was nothing to be concerned about.

I thought that maybe if I phrased my request in a different way, it would sink in. Yet she told me, in no uncertain terms, that there was nothing I could do about it.

At that point, I had a choice to make. Would I cower or stand up for what I believed—would I stand up for my daughter?

I chose the latter.

> *At that point, I had a choice to make.*
> *Would I cower or stand up for what I believed—*
> *would I stand up for my daughter?*
> *I chose the latter.*

Slowly and firmly I said that I didn't think she was hearing me correctly. If the resident stepped foot in Madison's room again, I would have my attorney here in five minutes. I would sue her, the resident, and the hospital.

This was something I never would have imagined myself saying before Madison got sick, but I had seen too much of the hospital staff not taking parents seriously. I was ready to do whatever it took to make sure that changed.

That night, I waited and waited to see what would happen, but the resident didn't come back to our room.

The next morning, I requested to see the resident's superior. I was glad my request had been honored that night, but I didn't want to risk having the entire issue buried. I had sat back while situations were swept under the rug before, but for this, I wasn't going to do it. I had felt the air change when that resident walked in the room, and I believed in my gut instinct. I was going to do what it took to make sure my child wasn't around that individual again. I was also going to voice what I thought about the resident being around anyone else's child.

Not long after I made the request, my husband and his family came to see us. While they were visiting with Madison, the head manager came by and asked if we could go somewhere to talk privately.

The family wanted to know what was going on, so I told them there were some events happening that I needed to bring attention to. As before, their response was kind but firm. They asked me not to make any problems in this place where Madison was being cared for. I saw their point of view; I really did understand. But I was there day in, day out. I saw things that they didn't, and I was not going to let anyone bully us anymore. Precisely because this was the place in charge of Madison's care, we needed to go to great lengths to make sure our voices were being heard and that patients—as well as their parents—were being respected. If I didn't stand up for them, for us, who would?

The manager and I found a private spot, and I immediately asked about the resident who came into our room. I did not mince words. She told me that many families had complained about him. While I wasn't surprised that there had been complaints, I was surprised that "many" families had encountered him. How "many" people had to complain before he was taken out of the rotation?

I asked why those parents hadn't been taken seriously. I wish I could say she had a good answer for me, but she didn't. I told her the severity I had felt in this situation and let her know I wasn't going to back down. If he set foot in our room again, I would move forward with a lawsuit.

A few days later, she came back to my room. She let me know that not only had the resident been removed from the floor, but he had also been moved into another role where he didn't have patient interaction.

I felt like this was a win—not just for the patients on our floor but for my own steps in learning how and when to speak up. The evidence was undeniable: following my gut was leading me in the right direction.

If the liver transplant was the biggest victory we'd had since coming into the hospital, Madison finishing her chemotherapy was a close second. There's a bell they keep in the cancer treatment area. When a patient is done with their treatments, they get to ring that bell. Madison wanted me to carry her. So together, on April 17, 2015, I walked her up to that bell, and she rang it. Everyone on the floor cheered, but Madison wasn't quite as excited as the others were. At this point, she just wanted to go home, to be a kid again and live her life. I couldn't blame her.

But I was so happy for her and also so proud. I'll never be able to get over the fact that such a young girl could summon the strength to go through all those treatments. As a mother, there was a part of me that also couldn't celebrate fully though. I was the one who had sat with her and saw her day in, day out—I sat beside her, holding her hand, watching what the chemotherapy did with my sweet little girl, how it made her so sick that she had her very own bucket to vomit in. Madison placed letters on it that spelled "PUKE BUCKET," and she used it for just that. For nearly ten months—maybe more; it felt endless—she vomited around the clock. Her stomach sickness was almost unbearable to handle and to clean up. A child shouldn't go through this, and a parent shouldn't be responsible for such heart-wrenching challenges.

It was pure pain watching her go through this. She was completely frail, withering away; her skin was dingy brown and muddy looking, skin colors I couldn't even recognize. Her smile was no more, and her face was sunken in. Every day, it felt like I was watching her die right in front of me. I would hold her little sixteen-pound frame in my arms and know how much healing we still had to do.

But what if I wasn't here for her? Who would take care of her? Who would clean her up every hour, every day, week after week when she was so sick from the chemotherapy, antibiotics, and steroids? My heart broke for those children who had no advocate, no one there to wipe their tears away and comfort them. Were their parents working, or were they just at home, thinking their children were being cared for. Or maybe it was a chosen separation because their child's pain was just too hard to handle or to watch? These questions filled my head . . . maybe more than they should have. But I knew the hospital didn't have the staff to offer these children part-time, let alone full-time, nurses. Those children were alone and cried every night; their screams and cries kept me stone sober as I sat awake night after night, researching and working.

It would be easier if there were more moments that were clear celebrations. But throughout this process, I was learning that everything "good" was both joy and pain. Relief lined with deep sadness. All these emotional lessons, though, were just a preliminary for the emotional tidal wave that was about to come.

It was Mother's Day when the wave hit. My friend Kim, who had been my trusted confidante, a day-in-day-out source of friendship, lost her daughter.

That her daughter died on Mother's Day is a fact I will never be able to get over. After such a long road lined with unfairness and heartbreak, to have that final twist of the knife in the heart for my friend was too much for me to even begin to comprehend. I was beside myself for Kim, beside myself for every mother who has gone through that experience.

As soon as I heard the news, I knew I would have to get out of the hospital, away from Madison. I hadn't been away from her for months, but I couldn't grieve for Kim next to Madison—that wouldn't be fair to her or to me.

From the moment I heard, I just kept thinking of Kim. The conversations we had. The struggles we had walked through together.

I'd always hoped *and* believed that we would both beat the odds and get our daughters well. After going through so much pain together, it only seemed right that we would go through their recovery together too. It wasn't God's plan though.

I was able to leave the hospital for one short evening. I couldn't think straight about where to go, so I ended up sitting by myself in a sushi restaurant, crying and reflecting. I felt guilty that my daughter was still here, but Kim had to say goodbye to her daughter. Kim and her family had to leave their little girl at the hospital and walk away empty and broken. I didn't know how she had the strength to do it.

I wanted to cry out to God to save Madison, but my faith was shaken to the core. I fought off the constant anger and doubt, wondering, *What did God expect us to feel after fighting for our children so hard, so faithfully, only to be left empty-handed at the end?* It wasn't fair! It simply wasn't fair. It was cruel, in fact.

I couldn't hold back my tears. I was certain everyone in the restaurant saw me. Who knows what they thought? A mother sitting alone in a restaurant, inconsolable, on Mother's Day. All I could think about was Kim and her family. How could I be there for her now? Could she still be there for me? Would it be fair to even expect her to be? My heart broke. I truly had no words or feelings left at this point. My faith was gone. I was at the lowest I had been thus far. The few things I thought were solid were gone too. Fear poured over me in that restaurant to the point that I couldn't breathe.

> *My heart broke. I truly had*
> *no words or feelings left at this point.*
> *My faith was gone. I was*
> *at the lowest I had been thus far.*

As I drove back to the hospital, I felt that I had lost my friend. How was I going to go on? How was she and her family supposed to go on? Our time in the hospital was always like this, surrounded by heart-wrenching questions there are no good answers to. You have to get good at sitting in the unknown, at learning to become very still while the storm swirls all around you, because there is no direction on where to go or what to do.

This was the beginning of a very dark time for me. Being so close to a mother who had lost her daughter put out my own inner light for a while. I don't know if anyone on the outside really sensed how deep this turning point was, but to me, I felt like I was only going through the motions of living. But I wasn't getting anywhere closer to the light at the end of the tunnel. Days turned into weeks and then months. We would go home for a couple of days only to end up back in the hospital because of "off" levels or a low-level illness Madison was fighting.

I had lost my job. And because my family didn't understand my fight for changes in the hospital, I sometimes felt like I had lost them. Hope was falling away. It wasn't all lost, but it was going fast.

The morphine didn't help.

We'd never known that Madison had an allergy to morphine until she was diagnosed. The first time she got morphine, she itched her skin like crazy for seventeen hours. It was unbearable to watch her clawing at an invisible predator— this relentless pain that only she could feel. There was nothing I could do, and I felt so hopeless. We were in the Pediatric Intensive Care Unit (PICU) alone, and it felt like no one was checking on us, that they'd all left us to wait it out alone. Her skin started bleeding, and she was screaming. I cried all night watching my daughter in agony.

The doctors said no more morphine, but then someone didn't check her chart, and she was administered morphine again. Once again, Madison went through hell.

After that mix-up, I started keeping my own notes in addition to what the hospital tracked. I recorded everything that went in her, with times and dosages. That was the information I used when the doctors tried to say her medicines didn't have contraindications. I took that list of what she had been taking and researched it. I was able to show them just how wrong they were. But they already knew they were wrong. I didn't really have to tell them.

Because I was always checking on what people were doing, I was able to stop a nurse who was trying to give Madison morphine—for a third time! She didn't even check Madison's ankle bracelet. I watched the whole situation unfolding. My internal warning bells started sounding, and I immediately asked what she was about to administer.

That woman looked at me and very calmly said, "Morphine."

To a child. Without looking at an allergy band. I almost lost my mind.

"*Get that morphine away from her,*" I yelled. And you better believe she did.

I called yet another meeting with the hospital administration about the incident. It was an emotional meeting; I just couldn't believe such negligence was happening.

Madison had me, and I knew other parents on the floor who were vigilant over their children. But what about the parents who couldn't be there watching every drug administered to their child because they were working every shift they could to pay medical bills. Or what about the kids who didn't have parents who wanted to be there.

Thinking about those kids put me into a spiral. One thought after another—everyone we encountered in this journey who had a story that had ended in pain. With thoughts like that haunting me, maybe it's not surprising that every day we were there gave me less and less hope.

Fewer reasons to believe Madison would ever get out so we could go home and be normal again.

Fewer reasons to believe we would be able to even say what was normal again. The storm was all we knew how to live in now. The hospital had become our home, more so than the outside world at that point. I felt deeply that we were too far gone.

Chapter Nine

PURPOSE IN THE STORM

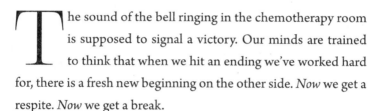

The sound of the bell ringing in the chemotherapy room is supposed to signal a victory. Our minds are trained to think that when we hit an ending we've worked hard for, there is a fresh new beginning on the other side. *Now* we get a respite. *Now* we get a break.

For Madison, nothing could have been further from the truth. Every time she jumped a hurdle—and, oh, the strength it took to get over each one of those hurdles—there was yet another hurdle for her to face, muster up courage for, and then get across. Getting a break? Or even a breather? Wishful thinking.

Right after she rang the bell, she got really sick. So they started pumping her full of steroids. The medicine load was huge, and all the steroids went into Madison through her PICC line.

PICC stands for peripherally inserted central catheter. It's a long, soft, flexible tube that gets inserted into a vein in the upper arm. They put a PICC in when a patient is going to be receiving lots of medicines and constantly finding a vein will be too hard.

When a PICC goes in, it stays in for at least a month at a time. You have to keep it dry and take care of it, and you're always watching to make sure there's no infection brewing around it.

So her PICC was in, and day in, day out, she was getting this massive amount of steroids. We would hook her up, and twenty-four hours a day it was running, and every forty-five minutes we were changing it. The steroids made her want to eat, which was a huge change from chemo. With chemo, she had no appetite, and nothing that went in could stay in. But very quickly after beginning steroids, she ballooned from sixteen pounds to fifty pounds. It was like she was going to bust out of her skin.

I was asking the doctors questions the whole time: Is this the only option? Are we sure this is helping her? Their answers were always the information they thought would pacify me, keep me out of the way, and keep me from bugging them with more questions.

> *Their answers were always the*
> *information they thought would pacify me,*
> *keep me out of the way, and keep me from*
> *bugging them with more questions.*

In my research, I had seen all the contraindications for the medicines they had her on, and I was taking those to the team. They insisted these medicines were necessary though, so I relented. The insinuation was that Madison needed these steroids if she wanted a fighting chance to get healthy. And the last thing I was going to do was put Madison in danger.

She did suffer hearing loss mainly due to those loads of steroids and antibiotics. Today she wears hearing aids and will for the rest of her life.

Those are the decisions and ramifications I still play back through my mind all the time. Did I do the right thing to let them keep her on those antibiotics and the chemotherapy? How does one decide between two potential evils?

When the hospital is always filling you with fear, it's so hard to say, "No, I have a gut feeling, and I'm going with that instead." I was fully committed to advocating for my daughter, but every day there was still that battle inside me. I was searching for the line . . . *how far is too far?*

I don't think it's too much of a stretch to say that no matter where we are in our lives, if we're standing up for what we love and believe in—whether that's people, our faith, a cause we are willing to sacrifice all for—there's that same question constantly being asked inside: *How far . . . how far . . . how far should I push it today . . . how far is too far?*

One thing Madison really had been looking forward to about ringing the bell at the end of chemo was that it meant she would finally get to make her wish. I'd always heard of Make-A-Wish and knew it was a great organization, but I had no idea the lengths they go to for these kids.

Immediately after she was done with chemo, we were given a Make-A-Wish family. At first it was strange to let this family into our house and our lives. We really weren't interacting with anyone who wasn't our own family or other parents in the hospital. There wasn't time to connect with others, and on top of that, emotionally, it was hard to relate to families who weren't dealing with what we were—and vice versa. But this family was so open and understanding. They were coming from this place of just wanting to help however they could. Once I saw that, it was easier for me to let down the walls I was living within 24/7 and let them in.

Madison was given the option of anything she wished for. Any trip. Any item. It was truly up to her. She didn't hesitate: Our sweet girl wanted to go to Disney!

Immediately, our sponsor family got to work on the trip. When a Make-A-Wish family goes to Disney, you get to stay on the grounds, and they set up every last detail. There's a limo that picks you up to take you to the airport, and the day before we left, they gifted Madison a party where she and a few friends were able to go to lunch and for a shopping spree at the Disney store. All her little friends came—the girls she had been in school with just a year before . . . even though, to us, it felt like more like a decade.

The girls had lunch at the Cheesecake Factory. I could tell they all felt so grown-up, ordering their favorite foods from those thick menus. At the Disney store, Madison got costumes—lots of costumes. And hairbrushes! Fifteen hairbrushes wouldn't have been enough for Madison; she just loved them. Her hair was growing back now that chemo was finished. I was praying she would never go through chemo again and lose that hair so she could use those brushes she loved so much!

After the mall trip, we went home, and she was so excited. I'll admit, I even got caught up in it. Here we were, finally done with chemotherapy. The day had been the most normal Madison had experienced in ages, just laughing with friends and having fun like every little girl should be able to. The next morning, we were leaving for a true family vacation, which loving people had put together for us. Without meaning to, I started to hope for this as our new beginning. Wishful thinking became *my* thinking: Could this be us going around the bend? Was a respite close? I didn't even care about a break for me; I just wanted it for my little girl.

When that little girl woke up the next morning to get ready for the limo that was on the way to pick her up, she had a fever.

No, no, no, this can't be happening. I was beside myself as I felt the heat on her forehead and recognized the familiar signs of sickness. The thermometer read 103 degrees. When I looked in her eyes, I could tell that she knew exactly what was happening. This was more than a fever. It was the end of the dream we'd all gotten sucked into. Normalcy wasn't an option. Breaks weren't coming. All the fun she'd had yesterday couldn't be her reality. It was so unfair! I could have raged against the world, but there wasn't time.

As soon as I called the hospital and told them Madison had a fever, they said she had to come in immediately. I knew what the answer to my next question would be, but couldn't help asking: "So we have to cancel her trip?"

The nurse I was talking to had compassion for me; she said, "I'm afraid so."

That's the world we were living in. Every time someone from the hospital took even one moment to acknowledge the hardship of what we were going through, it felt like a gift.

We called Make-A-Wish and told them what happened. I told them we had to cancel the trip. Even though they said we could reschedule at a later date, I just couldn't get far enough out of the disappointment to feel encouraged. All I could do was imagine that limo on the way to our house, then taking a U-turn. I felt that as it headed away from us, it took all our hope with it.

This was the beginning of when Madison didn't smile. The positive demeanor she had been holding on to slipped away, and she began to quietly withdraw. Every day that wore on in the hospital, with more tests and "off" levels and no definite date for leaving, felt like it took her further away from us. I kept wondering if we were ever going to get her back.

So many times, I had tried to put myself in her shoes, to imagine what it felt like for a four-year-old to be going through this, but I knew I couldn't imagine what it took for her to process all of it. We had been there for almost a year, and still, there was no end in sight.

Seeing Madison spiraling downward emotionally started to drain me in ways I hadn't yet experienced. I didn't realize how much her positive attitude was the encouragement I had needed to keep going.

Not long after Madison had been diagnosed, one of the nurses asked me if I could talk to a mother who had recently brought her child in. Her daughter was diagnosed with cancer, and she needed to speak to someone, to get encouragement that everything would be okay.

> *Seeing Madison spiraling downward emotionally started to drain me in ways I hadn't yet experienced. I didn't realize how much her positive attitude was the encouragement I had needed to keep going.*

I remember having absolutely no idea what I was going to tell this mother. Everything was so fresh then. The diagnosis had come only weeks before, and I could still feel tremors of that original storm rolling over us, changing our lives forever.

The day I talked to the other mother, Madison and I had been on our way out of the hospital. It was the first time we were allowed to leave. When I walked into the room where this mother stood beside her daughter lying in bed, through the doorway, I could see the elevator where Madison and I would be going next. It would have been so much easier just to leave the room and head for that elevator. But then I looked at Madison, and she smiled up at me with the sweetest smile. She was standing so close to me, like nothing could break her away. What could I say to this frail, crying mother, whose life had just turned upside down and been forever changed? I could tell her that nothing was more important than fighting with all her heart and soul for the daughter she loved.

I started talking to her, and even though I can't recall word-for-word what I said, I know the words gave that mother some peace, because I saw it come over her face. After we said goodbye and left the room and stood waiting for the elevator, I could hear the woman sobbing. It was such a mix of emotions. I was happy that Madison and I were walking out, but I was heartbroken for that mother who was terrified about this life she'd suddenly found herself in.

I heard the nurse, who meant well, tell the mother that everything would be okay. "Look at Amy and Madison. They are leaving today, and so will you."

In that moment, all the good feelings of having helped that mother fled my body, and chills went down my spine. I could feel it in my bones. I knew the truth about our leaving—it would be short-lived. And I realized how little help words from a stranger actually provide. They might give a little bump in mood for the moment, but it quickly fades as reality comes in around you.

That conversation still haunts me. Would I have encouraged the woman like I did if I knew Madison and I would still be there a year later? Madison's transplant had been successful, which was something to be so grateful for, but complications had continued. After so many months there, both of our mental states were worsening. Life was looking more and more hopeless. Madison was in a space where no one could say anything to encourage her, and I wasn't far behind.

People were trying their hardest to keep our spirits up. My grandmother sent me cards to encourage me. Every time Madison and I went home, we would find the letters on the cabinet waiting for us. These little notes represented so much love being sent across the miles, and that made a difference for me.

So often friends would reach out with brief texts or voicemails, just to let us know we were still remembered. But we knew. People forget. They move on. Life moves on for all of us.

And then of course, the evening visits from Eric and Zac kept me going.

But all that was only helping us hobble along; Eric and I sensed that all four of us needed something more. The disappointment of not taking the Make-A-Wish trip had deflated everyone too much. We decided everyone needed a break, and even if it took a lot of work to make it happen, we were going to take a vacation.

Puerto Vallarta, Mexico, was a quick flight away, and full of sunshine and beaches, which Madison loved. During a brief window of time that fall, when Madison was allowed to leave the hospital, we did it. We took that vacation.

The trip started out great and was so much of what we needed. But then a few days into the trip, Madison started to not feel so good. Instead of enjoying the beach and getting some healthy color from the sun, she slept for hours on end, the color left her skin, and her eyes took on a jaundiced look. We rushed back to the States and back to the hospital.

Once again, the doctors weren't happy with her levels— always it was talk of the levels. But this time around, they weren't willing to just do a scan to see what was going on with the levels. They wanted to do a liver biopsy.

There were risks with a biopsy, of course. Any time you have to go inside the body, there are going to be risks. The risks were minimal, but still, I wasn't crazy about the idea. Again though, when the doctors say there's no other way, it's hard not to let that sway you. And because there were no scans that could specifically check the liver, a biopsy was the only option we were given. I also think that because we had just been to Mexico, which I knew had pushed Madison's care team past their comfort zone, I felt like going along with the biopsy was what we needed to do.

I shouldn't have though. I should have stuck with my gut and insisted on just a scan. When they were inside Madison doing

180

this routine biopsy procedure, they nicked her transplanted liver, and the bile duct caved.

Normally livers have two bile ducts, but the liver Madison received was an adult liver that was portioned for two separate pediatric transplants, so she and the other transplant recipient each got one bile duct. So it was her only bile duct that had completely caved.

When the doctor came out of the room and told me what happened, I could hardly believe it. Literally, it was the worst news we could have received.

"What on earth do we do now?" I asked. I felt so desperate standing there, like my hands were tied behind my back, and there was nothing I could do to help my child.

The doctor said they would put her on drugs to see if they could do anything to slow the scarring process, which would render the bile duct incapable of reopening. He explained that once the bile ducts have caved even a little, it's very hard to get them to reopen and to get the blood to flow back through. If they couldn't get the duct to open, then the liver would be useless to Madison, and she would have to start back at square one. Looking for a new liver. Undergoing another transplant. The whole nine yards.

How does something like this happen?

What kind of surgeon nicks a liver in a routine biopsy?

Why did I ever let you talk me into this biopsy to begin with?

I was mad at her doctors, mad at myself, *mad at everyone.*

They said they wanted to do a year of stents, hoping that the stents would keep the bile duct propped open so that eventually blood would flow again. I didn't bother asking how likely that was though; I could see in their faces that the chances weren't great.

All of this together was just too much for Madison to take. Her demeanor went from withdrawn, the way she had been since the Make-A-Wish trip was canceled, to flat-out anger and rage. She was angry at everyone, and if I was being honest with myself, I couldn't blame her because I felt the same way.

Her moods were on a roller coaster, and I couldn't see the radical ups and downs coming. She would go into a rage, throwing things, screaming, telling me how much she hated me, and that all of this was my fault. She would demand that I leave the room until she called me back in. I had to push back the tears and sadness. I had to remind myself this was all very normal for a child who truly needed to release emotions that had been locked up in her for too long. She saw she was unable to change the situation no matter what she did. That wasn't just incomprehensible to her; it was unacceptable.

Whenever Madison woke up from a procedure, it was always hard. She had difficult transitions coming out of the anesthesia. During this time, however, it got even worse. Every time she woke up to find she was still hooked up to machines and stuck in a hospital, she went through every feeling of rage, anger, and frustration all over again.

After one procedure in particular, she woke up in a recovery room that we called the "glass room" because the walls were glass, so anybody walking by could see in. As soon as Madison woke up, she went into a rage. I felt that this rage was something different; the energy behind it was so desperate and angry. As it grew, she began to flail around in the bed, screaming at me and the machines—whatever she was staring at got her wrath.

She started pulling out the IVs. Then she stood up and pulled the phone out of the wall. I didn't know what to do. I felt frozen in place, and I felt an intense pressure inside my chest, like her little hand was inside squeezing my heart. I was beside myself; I felt broken. I knew why she was so angry, and I didn't blame her. There was also nothing I could do to help.

Nurses and residents walked by the room and looked in. They were watching the scene unfold—Madison so mad, me trying unsuccessfully to console her—and no one was doing anything to help! I felt like I was in a zoo, like we were caged animals to be observed. No one was empathizing with us, and no one was helping.

The weeks of trying to maneuver through Madison's anger had built up in me, so when I saw all those people watching yet ignoring what was happening, I snapped. I went out in the hallway, down to a waiting room, screaming, "No one cares!"

Both of us were out of our minds.

I called Eric. He had to come to stay with her. I just wasn't right, and I knew if I couldn't get a hold of myself, then I was never going to be able to help Madison in the ways she needed.

I do take comfort knowing that even when I was in a bad place, God had people in the right place to care for us. When we were in the muck of it, I couldn't always see His touch, but now, with the distance I have, I can look back and see so clearly where and how He was caring for Madison and me.

> *I do take comfort knowing*
> *that even when I was in a bad place,*
> *God had people in the right place*
> *to care for us.*

Barbie was a nurse who blessed Madison in so many ways. When Madison was really enraged, she wouldn't let nurses across the threshold into her room. Madison would growl and throw things at them. But with Barbie it was different. As soon as Madison caught sight of Barbie, it was like the tornado would start to wind down and then, after a few minutes of Barbie talking to her, she would actually be calm.

And Madison wasn't the only patient Barbie had that effect on. I think the other children saw and felt Barbie's true compassion for them.

I always wondered what it was that gave Barbie such a way with the children. Then one day, Barbie told me her sister died from a brain tumor when they were younger. The loss of her sister brought her to her "gift" of making very sick children feel very cared for. She vowed to go to school to become a nurse. I remember shedding some tears when she told me about her sister. Not only was I so sad for Barbie's loss, but I also recognized the truth about how fragile life is, and it really moved me. Why is it that we have to be broken by life before we can really understand how to help people put their own lives back together. When you are looking for people to care for your child, you realize how rare that skill is. Barbie was truly one in a million.

Not everyone has been through an experience like Barbie's sister or Madison, but at some point in our lives, we will all face hardships. At those times we will have to ask, How will I show up? What am I made of?

There were so many days I crashed and burned. After all, we are humans, and humans have bad days—especially under stressful, life-and-death situations. But I've come to believe it's how we bounce back from those hard times that truly matter. Now I care more about how I can pick myself up and how long it takes me to get back on track.

I spent the first few decades of my life wondering what my purpose was. I was always searching for it, like purpose was something you might suddenly find or stumble upon. I know I'm not the only one struggling to define that; just look at how many podcasts are out there promising purpose! Books line the bookstores! We are purpose-seeking people!

Even now, I'm not sure I know my purpose through and through, 100 percent. But this journey has gotten me a lot closer than I've ever been in my life. I think about Barbie and how she turned what was one of the hardest things in her life into a positive for so many people. *That's* worth living for. Learning how to find something to be thankful for every day, then being the thing that someone else is grateful for—*that's* purpose.

Those were some of the darkest days of my life. Hour to hour, minute to minute, I often didn't know how we were going to make it through. Fighting for Madison was always what kept me pushing forward though. I couldn't articulate that purpose yet, but it was all around me, swirling in the storm we were standing in the center of.

Chapter Ten

GOD, WE NEED
A MIRACLE

S tents were put in to encourage Madison's bile duct to open and let blood flow through it. The doctors, then, had to go in every four weeks to check the progress and to change them.

I don't know if you've ever been in a place in your life where you felt like things couldn't get worse . . . and then the floor dropped out another level. But this is where Madison and I were.

It seemed like nothing was going to change.

Like we were never going to escape the hospital.

Every *month* they were doing this major procedure, and in between them, we had test after test after test.

I was starting to believe the doctors were against us. And honestly, it doesn't feel like a stretch to say that. After all, this nick on the liver was a huge mistake, and it was all their doing. They continually ran tests and then came back to us after every round with results that always sounded so awful. And those awful results were always followed by with their orders to remain in the hospital. It was an uphill battle *not* to look at the relationship like it was us against them.

Every positive thing that had happened for Madison since we'd gotten in that place had either been due to her willpower and strength to fight through or because I had fought tooth and nail to advocate for her. I couldn't look around and see where any doctors were actively trying to help us. If it could be said that they were trying to help Madison get physically better, they definitely weren't doing what it would take to get her emotionally better.

For people who've never experienced something like this, it's easy to think that I'm overreacting or being too dramatic. I probably would have felt the same way had I and Madison not *lived* it. We never had a set schedule, but there was certainly a pattern to our lives then. With no say on our part, we would be required to stay in the hospital for at least four weeks at a time. And for seemingly no reason many of the times. Madison would be feeling fine, but the hospital protocol required running dozens of tests and seeing multiple teams regardless. It felt like they were just prolonging the exit strategy.

Unfortunately, during these stays, Madison would be climbing the walls. There was nothing for her to do but just wait and wait—for what? We never knew what we were waiting for. And then she'd get sick. Again. Whatever viruses or germs were making their rounds eventually found their way to her room, which required another two weeks of pumping her full of antibiotics, running more tests, performing more procedures . . .

I knew the only thing that would help her was time away from the hospital—time for her to try and feel like a normal little girl—but they weren't giving her that.

> *I knew the only thing that would help her*
> *was time away from the hospital—*
> *time for her to try and feel*
> *like a normal little girl—*
> *but they weren't giving her that.*

It's a dark place to be, in a system run by the doctors, while also feeling trapped by those doctors.

It's the kind of place that leads a person to . . . suicidal thoughts.

To dangerously speed down highways with your daughter in the back seat.

To feeling untethered in a way that makes you question if you were ever tied into anything in the first place.

To push the limits to see how low is low, how much God has forsaken you, or whether there is a shred of goodness left in the world.

The storm was swirling in me, and it was coming out in dangerous ways. Yelling "No one cares!" down the hospital halls was just the beginning. The kind of rage-filled episodes Madison was experiencing were beginning to hit me too, and with greater and greater frequency.

When I prayed, it was desperate and doubting. *Are You there, God? Are You watching this? Did You see her pull through that transplant only to have it all thrown into a delicate balance by the mistake of a surgeon? Did You see it happen during a "routine" procedure we didn't even want and didn't feel was necessary?*

Always when I prayed in the hospital, Madison would be in bed, and I would slip away and go over to my chair in the corner of the room. Hands clasped, head bowed, I would be on the floor talking to God.

For so long, I had prayed that God would heal Madison or that He would allow us to leave and be home in our beds, in the surroundings I knew could help us get healthy—if we could just get there. I believed those prayers had fallen on deaf ears though, and now I was over in that corner in the middle of the night, with tears on my face, the anger and rage bubbling up. The anger and rage were always there, my constant companions.

If I'm honest though, one thing was more prevalent than the anger: fear. It was everywhere. Every minute of every hour, fear was coursing through my veins. Being in a hospital that long, there were plenty of reasons to fear. But all the reasons really built up to my greatest fear of all—losing Madison.

Even when I wasn't letting that fear be at the front of my mind, it was still there. I was always resisting it, always trying to push it down. But here's the thing—I thought fear was bad. We're always told not to fear, that fear weakens us, that we need to stay away from it. But I've come to realize the truth. Fear itself isn't bad. It's bad if it freezes us and keeps us in one place, sure. But just having fear doesn't mean we're doing anything wrong. I think all my pushed-down fear was part of what made my emotions so hard to handle. I think it's part of what had me spinning out of control, flying down the highway, daring God to let my car spin out and take Madison and me out of our misery once and for all.

I saw my options as either giving into the fear and giving up or ignoring the fear so I could keep going. The fear was trying to keep me from the unknown. But I resisted it and said, "No, I have to go into the unknown for Madison to get better."

Looking back on that, the only thing I wonder is whether I should have considered a third option. What if I had embraced the fear? I wonder about that. I wonder if I could have saved myself that trip to the depths and the suicidal thoughts that had put me and my daughter in danger. What if I had used the fear as a tool that was on my side. Fuel to use up instead of a boundary to push against. Could the fear have actually helped me instead of hurt me?

That wasn't the way it was though. And I feel so lucky I found a way to get through those months when it was just getting darker and darker and darker. I've said it before, and I'll say it again: God was there, putting people in our lives, and making sure we had the skills we needed, when we needed them.

Grit is a word that is used in sales quite a bit. The top people in the organization—the sales reps who do the best—either they have it or they don't. I started out with grit, whether I was born with it, or I got it because I grew up in a situation where I had to create all my own opportunities. I think having grit was part of why I was drawn to sales. But then the longer I worked at it, and the more I understood what it took to be successful, the more that grit expanded and took root in who I am. For me, grit is determination and drive, the ability to push forward when you think you have absolutely nothing left to give.

I always knew God was pushing me toward developing more grit. But if I had stopped to think about it, I likely would have said He was doing it for professional reasons, so I could grow in my company and contribute more financial resources to our family.

Of course, after Madison got sick, it became so obvious. All that time, all my life, He'd been preparing me to stand firm through the hardest, most challenging situation I had ever faced. It truly amazes me how God uses experiences from all areas of life to do good things for His people!

In that particular moment in our lives, when both Madison and I were spiraling down, my grit was the only thing that kept us from getting sucked into the depths to a point we wouldn't be able to get out again.

I remember looking at my husband one night when he and Zac were at the hospital for dinner, and I told him I didn't know how much longer I could go on like this. He looked at me with compassion and empathy overflowing. He was hurting too, but to his credit, he didn't know what we were dealing with. The hospital was a whole other world of hurt.

He told me he would figure something out. I wanted to believe him. I desperately wanted to go back to a time when I could believe that kind of impossible and unknowable promise, when words could be like a blanket that I could just curl up beneath.

It wasn't that he had failed me; it was that everything and everyone had failed all of us.

That failure had taken my faith along with it.

As I recall, I couldn't even find words to respond to Eric when he made that promise.

If only I had known that very soon he would make it come true.

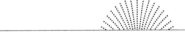

When your child is sick, it's hard not to want to believe in a miracle cure. I'm not one for schemes. "Get rich quick" schemes. "Get thin quick" schemes. All of that has always reeked of a hoax to me!

But any parent who has spent night after night with their child in a hospital bed would be telling lies if they didn't admit that they will at least turn their head and listen if someone starts talking about a miracle cure. Maybe they dismiss it after two seconds—once logic kicks in—but they at least get that sweet two seconds of believing there might be an easy way out of this hell.

> *But any parent who has spent night after night with their child in a hospital bed would be telling lies if they didn't admit that they will at least turn their head and listen if someone starts talking about a miracle cure.*

Eric is just like me. He's not going to believe in some kind of hoax. I know that we are both levelheaded people who aren't afraid to ask how real something can be if it sounds too good to be true.

Functional medicine. Holistic medicine. Alternative medicine. It goes by lots of names.

To some people, functional medicine sounds wishy-washy, something they should ignore. But there's so much evidence out there now—and now I've lived its truth—that it's hard for me to believe anybody would call it a hoax. Unfortunately, some still do.

We had been exposed to a type of holistic medicine back before Madison got sick. A good friend of ours, who was a chiropractor, would regularly give us adjustments. After the diagnosis, and when things got really bad with Madison, our friend asked Eric if we'd considered essential oils as a healing tool for her.

We had not considered essential oils. We'd never even *heard* of them. Our friend gave Eric the number of a representative for an essential oils company. The representative came to our house, sat in our kitchen, and told Eric what the oils could do. I wasn't there, but I trusted Eric to ask the right questions and make the correct decision. The oils weren't cheap. And they definitely weren't a guarantee, but they have been around for many years, they've been thoroughly researched, and they're known to be excellent for healing the organs. There was enough science there that Eric knew the oils weren't a hoax. And his gut feeling was that he needed to go for it.

After everything I'd been learning about going with my gut feeling, that was all I needed to hear. When he said he had invested in these things called essential oils and that we were going to start using them on Madison, I said okay. Considering we were pretty much at rock bottom, what more did we have to lose?

Along with the oils that Eric bought, the representative gave him two books, which contained all the information about the oils. I remember seeing those books for the first time and flipping through them casually. Little did I know that soon I would have many of the pages memorized! Or that it would get to the point where I so firmly believed in those oils that I always had one of the books with me no matter where I went.

I remember the first time Eric brought the oils and books

to the hospital. We had them all out and were looking at them. We were going to try three oils to start out. First was frankincense, which is especially good for cancer. The other two were for opening the bile duct, reducing inflammation, and increasing the body's ability to fight off infection.

The essential oils in their pure form are so intense that they will burn the skin, so they have to be mixed with V-6, a carrier oil blend that is safe to touch. Eric was telling me what the representative had taught him about the oils, and we were trying to get things together so we could apply them to Madison for the first time.

It's funny to think back to that day now. We were fumbling around, but it wasn't anxiety-filled or desperate, like so much of our time in the hospital had been. Even just getting the essential oils was a turning point for Eric, like he had been able to carve out a niche and really step up and help in a way that he couldn't when I was leading everything at the hospital. And as soon as he stepped up, I felt this mix of gratitude and relief, like I could let him take the wheel. There was something more too, something that's hard to put into words.

Had God heard us saying, "We can't do it alone anymore"? Were these essential oils His answer? I wasn't ready to voice any of that yet, but I had a stirring in my soul that said it was a possibility. And a stirring that pointed us somewhere—anywhere—other than darkness and depression and despair was *welcome*.

Madison was also interested in the oils. She wanted to

know all about them and what the possibilities were. That kind of spark from our girl was just what we wanted to see, and Eric was so ready to give her all the information she wanted. Seeing them connect was good. I thought that even if this was just something that pulled Madison from the place she'd been in—even just for a week or two—every penny *and more* would have been worth it.

As it ended up, we got that and so much more from the investment.

We started with the external mixture, placing it all over her liver area twice daily. It wasn't a huge amount, just a few drops. There was no way to really see if it was working. But her spirits were still up, and we were willing to do anything to keep that happening, so we invested in diffusers. First, for her room at home, then a small portable one for her hospital room. In our research, we had seen you could actually ingest them as well, but we didn't have capsules and the taste was so bad that we just stuck to diffusing it and putting it on her skin.

None of the hospital staff asked about the diffuser, and no one ever saw (or if they saw they didn't care to inquire about) me rubbing the oils on the area above Madison's liver. But we were diligent about it. Two applications a day, every day.

As I saw her attitude changing just with this small ray of hope, mine changed too. I started thinking a lot about defeat and our attitudes . . . and everything I've ever known and believed about how we can affect the outcomes in our lives.

Me—the woman who had always believed we make our

own destiny. How was it that I had somehow forgotten those words I lived by? Fear had been writing my story and making my destiny for months now. Maybe even all the way back to that first phone call I got from the school when they said Madison was sitting on the playground, fear was worming its way in, taking away my confidence, eroding my sense of purpose.

I realized I had to get hold of my attitude and change it. If I could get fear under control, then I could teach my daughter to do the same. We were going to have to believe in her healing for it to really happen.

So we started working on that.

I'm not a psychologist; I just have access to countless resources, and I keep my eyes open. I see, probably like you, how some people live feeling like they've won the lottery. And some people struggle along, like they got hit by a bus that day.

I've seen kids with their whole lives changed in a flash, relegated to hospital beds, taken away from their friends, yet who continue to have sweet and joyful spirits. And I've seen people living in mansions, with not a care in the world, with someone folding their socks, living like they can't catch a break, like everybody is out to get them.

I may not be able to believe anymore that we can completely change the outcome of our lives based on our hard work and attitude; seeing what Madison was going through had ripped that belief out of me. But I could absolutely believe that living a purposeful and rewarding life was all about how we approached whatever circumstances we were handed. Even if Madison wasn't old enough to fully understand that yet, I could show it to her by my example, an example she could hold on to for the rest of her life.

> *I could absolutely believe that living a purposeful and rewarding life was all about how we approached whatever circumstances we were handed.*

Every day when I was rubbing the oil on her, we would talk about fear. Openly. Honestly. We would talk about how we didn't have to give into fear—that we could fight it like the enemy it is.

We would talk about how encouraging others makes us feel good. How when feelings of despair come, if we let them take over, they can (quite literally in my case) take the wheel and then take over completely.

I didn't want Madison to be Pollyanna. We were still in a life-or-death battle, and I wasn't trying to diminish that at all. But I did want her to not feel so helpless and to know that even when it seemed like everything was out of our hands, there were still some factors we could control: our attitudes, how we loved the people around us, and how we loved God.

We couldn't control the outcomes of the monthly stent changes. But every month I would pray and pray and pray that *this* time they would see a change. The essential oils were helping emotionally; they were bolstering our faith and giving us the mental turnaround we had desperately needed. I knew that having a positive mindset would go a long way toward helping all of us. But part of me was really believing they could help physically too. However, the words from the doctor who told me that in all the years he'd been practicing medicine, he'd *never* seen a bile duct open and that we needed to prepare ourselves for another liver transplant, kept that fear alive in my mind.

The thing is, though, sometimes we just need encouragement, a way to get our emotions and our heads in a better, more positive space. The doctors' 100 percent guarantees of a negative outcome were never, ever helpful. Looking back, I see how the body fails under the pressure of negative promises, how it can manifest the very sickness that's "guaranteed." So many people stay much sicker than they have to be, all because they can't mentally pull themselves to a more positive place. I don't blame them. With all the "experts" speaking down to them, it's hard to believe in beating the odds.

We were doing our best to believe, but still, for months, there was no change.

Madison still had ten teams following her, which felt like ten million, and so the appointments and check-ins were constant.

Then, on top of that, there was monthly blood work, hearing scans for the damage done by the antibiotics and steroids, eyesight checks, and regular dental checks because of the risk of ill-development in the mouth and teeth. FAP can cause a small mark in the eye that looks like a little mole, so we also went to the eye doctor for that.

Madison had psychiatric evaluations that would go on and on and almost always ended with her in a meltdown. I'm all for the value of therapy, but most of those appointments felt like they were hurting a lot more than they helped.

The medical team even tested to see if she had learning disabilities.

With that constant rotation of appointments, even if we weren't checked into the hospital, she was always there.

Finally, in one of those meetings, I mentioned the essential oils. I was curious what the reaction would be, though I probably could have guessed. We were told to stop using the oils immediately. They were not FDA approved. We were told to stop everything we were doing that was above and beyond what the doctors ordered.

I paused in that room, unable to reconcile the tirade of warnings that had just rained down on me with the diffusing oils that filled the air in her room and the daily rituals that were such centering moments of calm and hope for us both.

Instead of reacting I listened to my gut.

These oils aren't deadly.

They don't come with two pages of dangers like every prescription drug they give us does.

201

And no one is willing to explain the dangers. They just want us to stop, while giving us no real explanation or reasoning.

I didn't lie and tell them we would stop. I just smiled and sat there and let them think what they were going to think. But I knew we weren't stopping. Who takes the one beacon of hope they have and smothers it under a sheet?

Not me. Their fear wasn't going to take root in me this time.

I will never forget the last stent change Madison had. At month twelve, the doctors were expecting nothing different; I could see it on their faces when we talked about the upcoming procedure. But I did what I always did. I sat out in that waiting room, praying and believing for something different.

The stakes were high. If there was no change this time, then Madison was going to need another transplant. But I couldn't stand by and watch her go under deadly anesthesia anymore! I was done with being treated like an experiment, a 100 percent guarantee that she would have another liver transplant, a 100 percent guarantee that she would get two more cancers. I needed a miracle. I needed God.

If there has ever been a time to show yourself, God, please let it be now.

I was thinking about how diligent we had been with the oils. How Eric had become such a part of the process through them. How discovering the oils had been this gateway toward us finding a shred of hope again. Emotionally, I wasn't fully better, but I had hope. And Madison and I were united in believing that we could overcome the fear of tomorrow.

When the doctor came out of that stent change his face was white as a sheet. He sat down before he spoke to me, which has never happened before. It was like he needed to catch his breath and gather his wits.

Looking back on the moment, maybe I should have panicked, but I had the opposite reaction. I knew in my gut what had happened. I felt the victory like the loudest, most resounding win of my life, like a crew of horses stampeding through the hospital.

"I've never seen anything like this in my life," he said. "It's healed. The liver is healed. The duct is open."

Then he stood up, walked away, and I never saw him again.

God used those essential oils to heal my daughter so she would not have to go through another liver transplant. I know that truth as solidly as I know the sky is blue and the earth is round. It was His deliverance in that situation, when we needed it most. *His faithfulness* is foundational for me. The only thing I wish is that I had my wits about me enough to explain to the surgeon what had happened. His scientific paradigm couldn't handle the mini miracle he had just seen.

Chapter Eleven

An Alternate Course

T he relief was immense. When that duct opened, it was like we all let out the breath we'd been holding for a year. For Eric, especially, it was a victory—his discovery of the essential oils had opened up the door of healing!

Of course, we weren't off the hook for all the testing they still wanted us to do, but we all could feel it—we had turned a corner. Madison was still frustrated at times, as I was too, but the edge was gone.

Before the duct opened, the possibilities of how bad the situation could get were always looming: *Will we have to do another transplant? Could the hell of the last year be just a warm-up?* Once it opened, we allowed ourselves to think about possibilities for how good the situation could get: *Will we be able to stay at home for long stretches of time? What if Madison can actually start school next fall?*

We got ourselves home as quickly as we could. They wanted us to stay for observation, but now that I'd seen how our intuition had been spot-on with the essential oils, I was so much more courageous about pushing for what I believed was best for Madison. I knew without a doubt, that girl needed to get home long enough to think of our house—and not the hospital—as her home.

The more research I'd done into essential oils, the more I'd started stumbling onto an increasing amount of information on functional medicine and clean living. I didn't have to investigate too long to see one of the first and most helpful things we could do was to start cleaning toxins out of our home. We started getting rid of plastics and reading *a lot* more ingredient labels. We were really focusing on Madison's nutrition—trying to make sure our food was less processed and heavy in fruits and veggies.

These changes were positive for all of us. While they were done with Madison in mind, in the end, I was a huge beneficiary of the efforts as well. With Madison finally feeling better, I never would have predicted sickness would be heading our way again soon. This time, it would be my own.

Spending so much time in hospitals, it was just impossible not to pick up whatever bugs were going around. I was too busy taking care of Madison to even think about taking care of myself. My doctors gave me antibiotics at first, but I still could never quite get completely healthy. It makes sense. I was tired, stressed, exposed to all those germs, barely able to exercise because we were always in the hospital, and we were living on food options they had there—which *weren't* healthy.

When the antibiotics didn't work, they added steroids. I had been sick for about eight months when Madison's bile duct opened. I finally came to grips with how sick I really was, probably because I was able to relax a little.

It was such a typical cycle for Western medicine: Patient is sick; give them drugs. Patient doesn't get better; give them a different kind of drug. When patient starts asking questions about why she isn't getting better, tell her you are doing everything you can do.

> *It was such a typical cycle for Western medicine:*
> *Patient is sick; give them drugs.*
> *Patient doesn't get better;*
> *give them a different kind of drug.*

I'd been seeing an ear, nose, and throat doctor (ENT) because, at first, I was diagnosed as having a sinus infection. The doctor suggested a surgery that could possibly help. I was so tired of feeling sick that I was willing to give it a try. One surgery became two, and in between, I ended up with a black fungal infection; black fungus forms were literally coming out of my sinuses.

I was so freaked out, I just kept going to the ENT. "What's happening to me?" I would ask. But he didn't know. He didn't know why surgeries hadn't worked and why I was still having horrible sinus issues. He had a guess of what to try for the fungal infection, but no guarantees.

207

After the second surgery, they put steroid packs up into my sinuses. Around the same time, I also got a staph infection. The infection traveled all through my sinuses and then my bloodstream. I think the doctors were scared for me. What had been bad suddenly was a whole lot worse. They took that opportunity to pass me off to infectious diseases.

I was so deathly sick and so exhausted, I couldn't get out of bed. The pain was still in the head and the sinuses and was moving into the chest. I was told the staph infection might eventually go dormant, but it would always be inside me.

There was a long list of all the unsuccessful antibiotics I'd been on, so when the new doctors said they wanted to put a PICC line in, I immediately asked what the heck they were planning to try through the line. It seemed to me we'd already tried everything! I handed the doctor the list of meds I had already taken, and I'll never forget his face while he read through it all. Finally, he sighed and said, "I don't know what you aren't completely intolerant to."

It sounded like a death sentence to me. "We're just going to get started putting more drugs in you and see what happens."

I was deteriorating so fast, there wasn't much hope. If I hadn't found Pat Bauer, I don't know what would have happened.

Pat was a godsend—I can say with 100 percent certainty, she saved my life.

An Alternate Course

Considering what our family had experienced with essential oils and the opening of Madison's bile duct, you'd think the first place I'd look when I got sick was functional medicine. But I didn't. I would say "old habits die hard" and shrug it off, but I think there is more to it.

For our whole lives, the idea of doctor superiority is hammered into our heads. We go to the doctor when we're sick, and if we want to get better, then we do what they tell us to do.

Even with my doubts about the Western medicine system—even after I'd spent so much time watching the system fail Madison—it was still my knee-jerk reaction to go there when I got sick.

Pat Bauer, an alternative medicine nurse, brought me back to my senses.

A friend recommended her to Eric, and when he told me about her, I figured I had nothing to lose. My alternative was to be hospitalized and become a guinea pig for Western medicine. I can say now, without a doubt, those experiments would have killed me!

Pat has gray, spiky hair, and she is as spunky as can be. She is kind and sweet. At first, she can be very quiet, perhaps because she's always observing and learning from the world around her. Where I had to practically beg the other doctors to give attention to my case, Pat was paying attention from the first moment of my first appointment with her. I found that as soon as you get her talking about what she's passionate about—health—she truly comes alive. Then she brings her patients to that place of vitality as well.

I shot straight with her. I told her everything that had been going on, that no one really knew what I was suffering from. I told her everything the doctors had done, so she would know how long I had been on antibiotics and steroids. I wanted to make sure she knew how dim the situation was.

She didn't hesitate in her response.

Very calmly she said, "I can help you." And something in me 100 percent believed her. It was the opposite of how I had been feeling for years—disappointed, fearful, ignored, treated like a nagging inconvenience. With Pat, I was secure that I was in good hands.

She squeezed me into her already booked-solid schedule, as a favor, and probably also because of the desperation and fear she likely heard when I first called her.

I was hopeful, but after all I had endured with what Madison went through, I also did keep something of a guard up. Still, even the most cynical patient could have felt encouraged around Pat. Finally, someone would talk about getting to the root of the problem—what I had been asking about for so long! She didn't just want to put a Band-Aid on it. And she sure wasn't telling me she couldn't help me with the hope that I would go pester someone else with my problems!

There was no saying that what I was experiencing was simply bad luck, and she *definitely* didn't leave me alone to cry and wonder in fear.

During that first conversation with her, I asked when she could possibly fit me in. Without hesitation, she told me she was fitting me in right now. There was no time to wait.

"Alright," I agreed. "Let's get started."

Ozone treatments can be a scary process at first because they are so new and foreign for most people. But Pat thought they were definitely the way for me to go, so she very carefully explained the process to me.

There's a gigantic bag that holds about 200 ml of your own blood. It takes a good amount of time to get it out. The blood then gets pumped through a machine where an ozone treatment kills the bad bacteria but keeps the good cells. After the blood comes out of the ozone machine, it's a raspberry color. It then goes through a red-light therapy machine before it goes back into your body. At that point, the good cells can start healing.

She explained that it would take multiple treatments, and every time you do a treatment it totally wipes you out. She wasn't kidding about that! After my first ozone treatment I went home and slept the rest of that day and through the night. Through that first treatment, I kept wondering, *Am I going to be okay?*

Pat said that following the second treatment, most patients can get back on their feet a little more quickly. But of course, everyone reacts differently, so there were no guarantees.

I had the opposite reaction of getting back on my feet. During the second treatment, I passed out. From what I was told, it happened pretty soon after the session began, and there was no waking me up. Their fear rose and rose until the office staff made the executive decision to call 911. An ambulance picked me up to take me to the hospital. During the ride, I vaguely remember waking up and not knowing where I was. I was confused, couldn't speak, and eventually passed out again.

When I finally woke up and saw Eric, I felt guilt wash over me. I had disturbed him during his workday, and I could tell that, although he was concerned about me, he needed to get back to work. I tried my hardest to fake it and act as if I was okay. The last thing I ever wanted to be was a burden to anyone. I'd been hearing Eric tell people for months now that things with our family were "great." People would ask how we were, and that's what he would say: "Everyone's doing great."

I wanted it to be true. But the truth was, I wasn't sure I was ever going to get better. After what we'd gone through, of course, I wanted everything to be great. But it wasn't, not with me. Nothing had been great for a long time, and certainly nothing was great now! I had this sickness I couldn't shake. Pat was the only person who had given me hope. But now I was torn between wanting to preserve this fake world of hope and the need to face reality.

> *I wanted everything to be great.*
> *But it wasn't, not with me.*
> *Nothing had been great for a long time,*
> *and certainly nothing was great now!*

At that point, I thought that perhaps I should turn back completely, give up on the alternative treatments, and go back to the traditional medicine that had up to then failed me.

I told Eric how I felt *emotionally*, scared and hopeless. But then we also discussed how I had felt better *physically* after the first treatment. He had done all the initial research and believed in what Pat was doing. And I did too. Ultimately, we decided I would keep going with the treatments.

I'm so glad we did. When I went back for the third treatment, it was life-changing. That was the moment everything turned around for me—I felt tired, but I felt so much better overall.

When I was originally researching ozone treatments, I had reached out to my ENT doctor to ask him about them. He told me they were voodoo, and I absolutely should not touch them. However, by the time I was through two cycles, I was like a brand-new woman. I printed out all kinds of clinical data on ozone treatments and took them to his office. I handed the information to the nurse with a little note that encouraged the doctor to consider educating himself on alternatives *that are saving people's lives.*

I also took the clinical data to my infectious disease doctor. He was more open-minded. I saw him when I was on the mend, and I said to him, "If these halls were wider, I would be doing cartwheels. That's how great I feel."

His eyes were as wide as saucers! The doctor said, "I don't

know what you're doing, but keep with it because I've never seen a patient come back like this from what you had."

And come back, I did! Over a six-month timeframe, I had about fifteen treatments. At that point, Pat tested me for the staph the doctors said would always lay dormant in my system. It was completely gone! The staph was completely eliminated from my body!

I knew I couldn't make those doctors read or care about that clinical information. But I have always hoped they did, not because I live in an alternate reality where I think patients can convince doctors to change their minds. But it's my hope that maybe—just maybe—if another patient came along and asked about alternative treatment options, they might respond at least a little differently than they did to me.

It took well over a year, a long list of dietary changes, and working out some major mental blocks for the complete turnaround. But I eventually went from barely being able to get out of bed, with no idea why and no one able to give me answers, to being healthier than I'd been since I was a little kid.

My energy was high.

Vitality was coursing through my body.

The change was so pronounced that almost everyone I knew, after just one look, at some point asked what was going on with me.

Isn't that interesting? It's such a statement of our healthcare system as it is today: When people are actually, truly healthy, it stands out so much that others want to know *how* it's happened!

Every time anyone asks, I slow down and tell them our experience, from the first discovery of essential oils to my ozone treatments, which wiped out the staph infection, to the vitamin infusions I now take. It's not enough to say, "It's functional medicine." That's such a huge net to cast; even if someone wanted to look into an alternate way of caring for themselves, how could they start with that?

I tell them our experience. I don't leave out the wrong turns we took or the hiccups we had. I never tell anyone that going against the grain is easy. I don't want them to think, when they hit the first bump, that it's not for them. I truly believe it's lifesaving— it was for us. So I want people to not just explore how functional medicine can better their lives, but I want them to actually take steps toward making health and true wellness their reality!

After seeing all the changes in my health, we wanted even more assistance for Madison. I wasn't going to stop advocating for her, and I intended to get Madison the best options in functional medicine! I wanted Madison's body to be as healthy as possible, to possibly dodge this 100 percent guarantee of a second and third cancer due to her rare FAP gene. Nothing could stop me from looking at every possible option for my little girl! I wouldn't be able to live with myself if I didn't push the limits and defy the odds stacked against us.

Pat Bauer didn't work with children, only people seventeen years and up, so we began searching for someone who did. We followed every lead given to us but with no luck. Functional medicine practitioners for children are in high demand, but they fly under the radar, seemingly afraid they will be "called out" for treating children using non-FDA approved options. What most people may not be aware of is that FDA backs what makes the most money: treatments that don't consistently cure but do bring in money for hospitals and medical companies—and that consistently keep people sick!

While we researched possibilities for Madison's care, Pat kept giving us great leads. She told us about Hope for Cancer in Mexico. I reached out to them and got lots of great information. She also told us about Dr. James, who was in the process of setting up her practice. She eventually moved into Pat's building and opened up a pediatric practice. Dr. James was offering IV infusion therapy, orthopedic care, pediatric care, urgent care, and ozone treatment with red-light therapy, and hyperbaric oxygen treatments. In 2021, she treated Madison with IV infusions, and we discussed Madison's case thoroughly. Should any of Madison's cancer return, Dr. James is who we would work with.

We needed a holistic approach to Madison's general care too, though. We were finally referred to one of the best in the business, or at least here in the Midwest. Until the time of this writing (2023), this doctor couldn't be found by an internet search or through social media. Word of mouth was it! Dr. Scott

Huff came with the highest recommendations for offering patients something that was quite rare in health care—a deep dive into your care.

Dr. Huff's approach is to teach patients how to develop a relationship with their body, to understand what's going in, how all the systems work together, and how the body is being cared for in *every facet of interactions.*

His care for Madison began by helping her and our entire family look—and truly see—how our lifestyle and habits might be adversely affecting our health. He taught us about internal and external toxins, how certain lifestyle factors play into the bigger picture, what an acidic environment means and how it's created, and how each of us can be affected by heavy metals, molds, inflammation, microbes, and stressors that affect the body, such as allergies, foods, etc.

It was a huge, perspective-shifting first step, and it was just the beginning!

It's one thing to say it, but another to truly understand that, to achieve optimal health, we must change our mindset, nutrition, lifestyle, and environment. We must increase the body's tolerance and do more extensive lab testing so we can understand what's happening inside us and can better fortify our bodies to resist attack from the environmental factors that are outside of our control.

There are some cancer drugs that have merit, but they treat the cancer; they don't treat *you.* And after cancer has been diagnosed, it can be too late. With Dr. Huff, we made a plan to treat all of our bodies and correct our lifestyles *before* cancer strikes.

> *It's one thing to say it, but another*
> *to truly understand that, to achieve optimal health,*
> *we must change our mindset, nutrition,*
> *lifestyle, and environment.*

Thanks to him, we look at everything different now.

The genetics doctors say more cancer is coming for Madison, but I am bound and determined to prove them wrong. I know that finding Madison a functional medicine physician was the first and most important step.

As for my health, I wish I'd never gotten stuck in that cycle of steroids and antibiotics. At the same time, I know I did what I had to do. To focus on Madison required perseverance. I wouldn't change my role as her primary caretaker for anything. But eventually, I had to figure out how to get myself healthy, so I could help my family with their health.

I look back and see so many points at which I could have made different and better decisions. For so long after Madison got sick, I was chasing the wrong things. I was trying to figure out "why" when the right question was "what's best for my daughter now?" I wanted to control the situation, and I was searching through my past, for what I had done wrong, medications I took before and during pregnancy, vaccines, or shots the kids had. I thought if I could figure out the root of the problem, *then* it would be manageable.

The pediatrician my kids had seen since birth was so upset by our questions about vaccines that we were fired from the practice. We were sent a letter asking us not to come back. I can go back and see myself sitting in so many doctors' offices asking questions, getting blank stares, or being ignored completely. It was a lonely road to walk, which started with my decision not to go along with whatever we were told but to advocate for my daughter.

There was a learning curve.

Sometimes I pushed too hard, other times not enough.

So many tears were shed, so many sleepless nights endured as I armed myself with information.

When a person challenges "the way things are" they will be bullied, questioned, and threatened. But are any of those good reasons to step off the course? To back down?

I'm not going to lie, there were moments when I felt weak. But then I would see my daughter, or I would find myself on my knees, asking God what to do next. And I would find the strength to continue with what I had to do to get her—and then myself—well.

Chapter Twelve

It is Never Wrong to Advocate for Yourself

When I was sixteen, Chad went to jail. Sadly, at that point, it wasn't surprising at all. My brother had already been there a couple of times before. But what was new *this* time was that he used his one phone call to call me. As soon as I answered the phone and accepted the operator's request to pay for the charges, he asked if I would do something for him. I had the immediate urge to say no but I said yes. I had such a strong pull toward him, and maybe I still believed that things would turn around and go back to how they used to be—our family, happy; the two of us, best friends; and us riding around in his truck listening to music, telling jokes—all the good days I missed so terribly.

I asked him what he needed me to do.

He gave me directions to a house in town. He had hidden money in the ceiling. He instructed me to go to this house, find the one specific ceiling square in a closet, push it up and out of

221

the way, then rummage around until I found a bag of money. I was then to sneak it out of the house when I left.

It was the craziest thing anyone had ever asked of me. But this was my only brother. I didn't think about myself or what was right or safe. I told him I would do it.

Within the hour I had driven myself over to the house and told the person who answered that my brother had left something inside. They let me in, which is in itself strange. But what I was doing was actually the strangest part. I made my way to the closet and felt all around that ceiling square—of a house I didn't know!

The money was gone, though, which doesn't surprise me. I've often wondered if that's why those people let me into their home to dig around in their ceiling of all places! They had already found the money and taken it for themselves. The easiest way for Chad to know he was never getting it back was to let his sister see for herself that it was gone.

Regardless of anyone's intentions, when I was driving home from that house it slowly dawned on me how dangerous that whole situation had been. For sure the money had come from some kind of illegal activity. The people living in that house were drug users in some way, shape, or fashion; my brother had pretty much exclusively hung out with people who did drugs too. It would have been all too easy for someone on a whim to decide I looked out of place or to get a funny feeling about me and then pull a gun.

Going into that house was the most dangerous thing I had ever done. And now I had to come to terms with the fact that my brother had asked it of me.

Every day, I watched my parents set aside all logic so they could take coddle my brother and allow his destructive lifestyle to continue. Was I going to be a part of that, or was I going to look out for myself, become an advocate for what I needed to do for my own life, and go my own way? Of course, at the time I could never have guessed that this would be a training ground for later in life when I would face the same questions: Would I step up and protect my child and myself? Did I have the courage to push against the pressures facing us so I could put us first?

After going into that house that day, I decided I was ready to advocate for myself. And for the rest of my life, I never gave in to a request that put me in a precarious or dangerous situation. It was a breaking point for me. But it was also one for Chad and my parents, because I was really drawing a line in the sand declaring who I was going to be and how I was going to live. It had to be done. And I've never once regretted it.

Not long ago my brother and I sat down to talk about the past and where we are today. Our lives have always been on two different trajectories, but we had never put words to it nor shared the thought with each other. It was one of those conversations that had never been had.

Chad has spent his life in and out of prison, never having a steady job, home, or family, and he has lost custody of his many

223

children. Yet he seems to believe every decision he ever made was exactly how he wanted his life.

For years, I had been beyond frustrated, watching how my parents continued the cycle of giving to him while he abused their love. Even when he would break into their home to take money or their belongings to pawn, they would *always* welcome him back. They would continue to give and give and give, both emotionally and financially. Just sitting by and watching was too much for me to take, especially when I felt like my own children weren't getting their attention because it all went to Chad.

My mother had always wanted us to put on a happy face for the holidays. For many years, we went along with the charade. We would be trying to enjoy the day together, and Chad would show up, monopolize the conversation, take his presents and their money, then disappear. He would pop up only when it was time, yet again, to get bailed out of prison.

Finally, I decided it was too much sitting through the lie of a happy holiday on what was supposed to be the happiest day of the year. A few years ago, when I found out my brother was once again at my parents' house, with who-knows-what characters he brought, I went to him directly. I told him I never wanted him to contact me again, that I would not condone what he had done to our parents, and how he would show up every time he was out of prison, drop into our lives or onto their doorstep, and act like nothing had occurred.

Chad was furious. He bit back with a vengeance and told

me that I knew nothing about his life or what he had or hadn't done.

After that conversation I truly didn't think he and I would ever speak again. I was filled with rage and could tell he was too. After so many decades of wishing my family could be healthy and happy, I was exhausted. It was easier to walk away than watch any more emotional energy get sucked up by his life and choices.

But then that day came not long ago, when we both ended up in a place where we could talk without ripping each other's throats out. As we communicated for the first time in so many years, I came to an understanding I'd never had before. When I made that decision at sixteen to keep myself safe, I was choosing how I was going to live. And even if I don't agree with my brother's choices, all of them were coming from that same desire: to steer his own ship.

During that conversation, I realized the acceptance I have kept from him for all these decades is the exact same acceptance I want from others. As I am choosing to challenge authority, push against rules, and dig for a better way of doing things, I want to be able to be free to live my life as I want—even if others think it's not appropriate. Once I saw *acceptance* in this way, I could look through my life and see how I needed to start handing out that kind of freedom to others.

As Zac gets older and needs more and more independence, I need to step back so he has the room he needs to fly.

Eric has started another business that requires an entirely

new skill set, and I need to let him explore that, with all of its ups and downs, on his own. The part of me who wants to micromanage needs to shut down.

I think back to how I felt when Madison started school, after years of being in the hospital and being homeschooled. I'd been with her every day for so long, but now I had to let go. And I had to accept how she wanted to approach this challenge of being a regular kid in a regular school.

I'm not saying I need to be passive in the lives of the people I love. I still want to bring my opinions, and hopefully my help, so that I can enhance their lives. Especially for my children, I very much will remain a guiding force as long as they are home with us. It's just that, for the first time, I realize I must be myself and advocate for them in big and small ways every day. So they can find their own voices and their own ways through the world. Most importantly, so they can grow into advocates for themselves. But while I'm doing that, I also must understand that I can't control the decisions they make or the outcome of those decisions.

It's not an easy balance to strike! The easier way is to steamroll through and try to make it my way or the highway. But if I do it that way, they will all get the life I want for them, not the life they want. Considering the last years that we have all fought so hard for, I want every day to be a move toward the space where they thrive.

Does that sound strange? Maybe. But think about how many people we know who aren't really living their lives, who are locked up by fear or past choices or what they think they should do instead of what they are born to do. Or locked up by unforgiveness.

Through all this, I have learned that in forgiveness, we have true freedom. Freedom, not just so we can decide to go our own way. But the kind of freedom that gives us assurance that our hearts are clear so we can follow God's way, so we can sense those little nudges that He gives all of us.

> *Through all this, I have learned that in forgiveness, we have true freedom.*

I believe that's the only way to really live life to the fullest. Any day and every day I want to be advocating for where I hear and feel God's call on my life. And I want to help people around me do the same.

What about you?

Chapter Thirteen

EXIT STRATEGY

A few months ago, I splurged and bought myself a new desk. For twenty years, I'd been using the same desk, and it was time. Before the new desk was delivered, I started going through the drawers of the old one so I could get organized.

While cleaning it out, I found a large envelope. My heart stopped when I opened it. It wasn't just a stack of hospital forms like the ones I'd been combing through for the last hour—this was my half-written letter to the family of the organ donor who had saved my daughter's life. The letter fell into my lap along with photos of Madison—photos I didn't even remember we had taken! I thought I had sent this nine years ago! Why had it been forgotten and shoved in a drawer? How come I couldn't remember finishing it, let alone stashing it away? The only answer was that I was so broken then and was living in such a haze. It must have hurt more than I could handle to even write the words.

The letter wasn't finished, and as I read back through each

painstaking line—some of them scrawled out so jaggedly it seemed as though I had been crying while I wrote—I could sense the struggle I had with every word. The person I was when I wrote that letter started coming back to me. I was so lost and broken, tortured by what my daughter was going through. Every day, there was such a strong pull toward sickness and fear; the force of fighting against it had literally drained the life from me.

Looking back from that perspective, I think maybe that's why I didn't send the letter. Perhaps it was too painful. It was clear to me that I had felt really torn up over what to even say; the letter jumped all around, and some of the ideas I was trying to convey didn't make sense.

Even though I can remember the woman I was, the idea of going back and living through that again is too much to bear.

So much has changed for me since then. Physically. Emotionally. Spiritually. I'm a new woman.

And the change isn't done yet. God is healing me . . . my heart is healing.

Holding that letter in my hand, I knew without a doubt, God was telling me that now was the time to finish it. This time, as I wrote, the words came out of me so easily. I put the original photos back in the envelope, but I also added more recent ones so they could see the woman Madison is growing up to be. It's the life made possible by their unimaginable loss.

This time, as soon as I finished the letter, I sent it. I don't know if I will ever hear back from the family but that wasn't the point. I just needed them to know how grateful we are. I also needed to see that now I could write the letter as it needed to be *and* that I could send it. Proof I am moving forward. (Even though God is the one who has been doing all the moving!)

When Madison was finally out of the hospital for an extended period of time, and we felt like we were living in the world again, I would get so frustrated when I saw others get upset over the littlest things, things I saw as simple challenges. We had been through way worse! I would have to fight to keep from saying, "Oh my goodness gracious, stop your crying!"

The chip on my shoulder was extra large, and I had a huge attitude to get over. Time was a big part of getting past it, but there's a grace piece too. So I took it to God.

Since I found Him again in that hospital, I have never stopped praying. I always find Him. My favorite place to seek God is in the outdoors. I see Him in the trees and in the birds. When I am surrounded by nature, I feel surrounded by Him.

In all those moments, He's nudging me forward. Sometimes the changes are so small, I can't see them. But when I look back and see the miles covered, I am so grateful!

Since we left the hospital, there have been a handful of times when I have felt drawn to the park that we used to be able to see from Madison's window. When I am in that outdoor space, feeling God all around me, I look up to that hospital and think about the people I knew there. I think about the lifelines who got us through—Barbie, Kim, all the mothers and fathers I would stand silently with in the hallways while we drank our coffees and tried to hold ourselves together. Often, I say to people, when you drive by the hospital, look up. There are people in there who never get to leave.

> *My favorite place to seek God is in the outdoors.*
> *I see Him in the trees and in the birds.*
> *When I am surrounded by nature,*
> *I feel surrounded by Him.*

It's not my reality anymore, and I am so grateful for that, but I know the truth is that even when we stopped being long-term residents of the hospital, I left a little part of myself there. Madison and I are on the same page with having to heal what the years in the hospital took from us. I tell her—and myself—that we have to give ourselves grace, that it can't be a quick, overnight process to get rid of the anger, hurt, and defensiveness. But there is no skipping that work! It must be done; we must get healthy on the inside. There is power in positivity—in thinking positively, which is something we've done much more of over the last several years.

For a long time after we got out of the hospital, Madison would freak out if we even drove by. The mention of it could send her into an emotional spiral. I understood it completely—the closer she got toward a normal life, the more fearful she would become of watching all the normalcy be snatched away again. None of us have those answers about tomorrow though;

there are no guarantees. All we have control over is the day we are in right now.

It's our choice to live it without fear.

I say it to her. I say it to myself. Over and over again.

It's scary to see the steps she takes backward when she goes for the yearly checkups or to get blood drawn. I don't know if in those times, she will ever be able to completely chase away the fear—it hits too close to the cancer she already beat once, especially the blood work. When she does those tests, she always spends the next day asking, "Did you get the results? Did you get the results?"

The doctors called after the blood work last time. They said things were off. They wanted to increase her doses of medicine. They also wanted to redo labs as soon as possible, but I pushed back. I felt that if we start adjusting doses, then I'm worried it will mess her up, and she'll be stuck in the cycle of needing more and more blood work, which always comes back "off," and slowly we will slide back toward the hospital.

In the beginning, I never would have given the doctors a definitive no. I was never comfortable enough to define our own boundaries. But a year ago we did it—we said, "No, I think we are going to do labs every three months."

We had to have those three months in between tests. Otherwise, the cycle of fear would start moving back in on us. Then, when they let us stick with three months, I got bold and said, "I think we'll push it to every six months."

They went along with it for about a year and a half!

At that point, I started asking about the exit strategy. How long were they planning to test Madison? When could we quit altogether? When I asked, I could see on their faces they wanted us to stay with it indefinitely, but luckily those weren't the only experts I could turn to. I had found alternatives to simply testing and waiting for sickness to strike again.

We were so lucky to find Dr. Scott Huff, who works with us on a monthly basis to keep Madison's body physically healthy.

He took us on a deep dive that is changing and will forever change our lives. He began adjusting even more of her diet, really digging into removing all toxins from our home, and continuing to focus even more on the power of the positive mind frame, not letting the negative thoughts take control.

Dr. Huff also was the doctor who finally gave me the answer I'd been frantically searching for at the beginning of this journey, when I was haunted by the question: Where did this cancer come from?

Dr. Huff said there was not one root event that started it all. "Instead," he said to me, "it was a perfect storm."

A "perfect storm" of what? As Eric and I have dug into all these things and have learned so much over the years, we see it as a combination of all sorts of things: gut health, lifestyle stress, food and environmental toxins, bad air quality, medications or vaccines, the list is endless.

Ever since he said that to me, I have so often pictured

Madison and me walking out of the storm together. From tormenting rains, dark skies, lightning, and thunder that makes you jump—into dry land, with the sun shining, and peaceful skies.

The cancer might still be out there, I can't say for sure we won't ever walk back into the storm. But as for today . . . I choose to live without fear. That's what I keep saying: "Today, all is well."

> *But as for today . . .*
> *I choose to live without fear.*
> *That's what I keep saying:*
> *"Today, all is well."*

Reminding myself of that is a daily practice. Even after this time I've spent working hard at it, there's nothing automatic to it.

For years and years, after we were back home, I was angry—so angry!

I was angry at Eric that he wasn't in the hospital with us all the time.

I was angry at complete strangers.

Sometimes I would still get angry at God.

I'd wake up angry and go to bed angry.

Sometimes I was so angry I would just cry—I've cried more in the last five years than I ever cried going through the actual sickness with Madison. Guilt, shame, picking fights with Eric. It was always something. I would always be mad at something. He would always be doing something wrong.

Then one morning after I dropped Madison off at school, I don't know what came over me—it was like I was being physically pulled toward the church that's above her school. I parked my car because, honestly, I didn't even feel like I had a choice.

I was living in this complete and utter nightmare again. Even though Madison was good! She was well! Still, all those negative feelings were coming up in me. I was trying to push them away with positive talk, which sometimes worked . . . for a time. But fundamentally, foundationally, my heart had not changed. I was without fear for the day, but something deeper was off—I was still carrying around too much rage.

I think God had been going along with me, but He finally got to a point where He was like, "She is just not getting it. I'm going to have to drag her into a church so she will surrender."

I went into the main sanctuary and sat there for the longest time. No one came in;, no one asked me to leave. I just prayed to God that He would heal me. That He would somehow bring calmness, somehow bring healing. He was trying to do something in me, and I couldn't figure it out.

But that was the moment the storm was thrashing around—giving one last fight before the final clearing. The way I dragged myself into that church and laid myself before the Lord to let whatever was to come just come. It was like giving birth, a process you have to hand yourself over to. All you know is the pain, but there's no way around it. All I was clinging to was faith that He would get me to the other side.

When I left the church, I felt wiped out, and for weeks, I walked around in a daze. Eric kept asking if I was okay. And I was. I just felt like I was really deep in my thoughts, like I was walking with God.

Over and over again, I thought about that day so many years ago when I was speeding down the highway, with Madison in her car seat and suicidal thoughts in my head. The memory of that day kept growing further and further away. It was like God was making it fuzzy and taking away the teeth of those feelings so they couldn't get me anymore.

In my mind, my foot wasn't on the accelerator or on the brake. God Himself was guiding the car; He was taking me to the next step. I couldn't do it on my own; He was helping me.

I remembered the question I had regularly asked myself and others all through that time: How do we prepare for what is inevitable?

It's not *if* tragedy and heartbreak will find you, but *when*. That's part of being human. Our feet will press too hard on the gas; we will end up out of control.

When our world was coming down around us, I was always wishing for a guidebook. But now I am so glad no one handed it to me. I remember sitting in that hospital room day after day, then weeks and months . . . I would look out the closest window while I prayed— begged, really—for forgiveness, answers, guidance, calmness.

But now, years later, God was giving me such a gift. He was handing me grace. I gave Him the guilt, the anger, the regret, the rage. I stayed in constant conversation with Him about my daughter, my son, and my husband. I asked that we could all continue to heal.

I was walking around in a daze, because He was showing me that the way to see *everything* is through Him. I can always write my story with God And it's not one of self-reliance; it's a story of reliance on Him, His ways, His timing, His plan.

When that fog began to clear, my heart was clear in a way I hadn't felt in so, so long. The storm was diminishing. The land was drying. I could see and welcome the sun. The skies were beginning to show peace.

My daughter was well, and finally, I felt a glimmer of hope that I hadn't felt in over nine years, when life was good, without fear, without extreme sadness and destruction.

Now I know what it is to advocate for someone, to put everything I have into something outside of myself. Without advocating for Madison, I never would have found this deep and passionate relationship with God because I never would have needed Him so desperately.

We have to lose ourselves to find ourselves in Him. I'd heard it so many times, but now I understood it.

So I want to leave you with the most difficult questions yet: How will you advocate in your life? What will you fight for? What will it look like?

For two decades, I was in my own way, always looking for my gifts and purpose. If I'd shifted the focus from me, me, me and what *my* purpose was, maybe it would have allowed more space for God to move.

Because He is always moving. That's one thing I know with every fiber of my body. Even in—no—*especially* in the middle of a storm.

EPILOGUE

This story is about my daughter's cancer, how it changed us and ripped us apart, and it's about how we finally let God in to heal us. It's about how I learned to be an advocate.

In learning to be an advocate, I could look back through my life and see that all along, God was giving me the tools I needed for that advocacy—that He was always preparing the fighter in me, so that when the storm came, I could weather it.

My prayer is that you and your family will never go through an ordeal like ours. After the years I spent meeting so many families who were living through the same hell as we were, I very sadly am aware that it does happen to more people than any of us want to imagine.

Whether you are fighting an illness for yourself or a loved one, or you are in a different life battle altogether—all of us can become better advocates for ourselves and the people who matter most to us.

We can research the heck out of whatever is in front of us and look at the problem from all kinds of angles.

We can ask questions when things don't make sense or feel right.

We can listen to our intuition.

We can cry out to God and listen to what He has to say.

Then we can act on what we learn.

We can stand up for ourselves and what we know is our best path forward.

We can't control the future; we can't keep the storms from coming. But we sure can choose how we make our way through the rains.

Every day we have the choice to live without fear.

As I was finishing this book, we got a call from Madison's team at the hospital. They were letting us know that they want to start screening her for thyroid cancer. That's the third cancer her genetic tests revealed. She already gets screened for the colon cancer that they predicted would come around age thirteen (which is around the corner). She's also going to be regularly tested for the one that's supposed to arrive in her late thirties.

All of the unknowns involved in that testing are enough to drive a person mad. But I'll say it again . . .

Every day.

Epilogue

We have the choice.

To live without fear.

A few years ago, Madison started doing acro gymnastics. If you've never heard of it, look it up. Then imagine a petite, beautiful, young warrior woman literally flying through the air.

Perhaps it should be no surprise, but she has incredible physical strength for a girl of her size. Paired with the intense determination she forged in the flames of her illness, it's phenomenal to watch what she can do.

Sometimes when I watch her, I get lost in the sheer joy of watching her in the middle of all that freedom. Isn't that what we all are wishing for? To be able to live so free?

Even after all we have been through, I believe freedom is still out there. Some days I feel it so fully. I am unrestrained, walking the imperfect, painful, and glorious path God intended for me. May you have moments of such freedom too, friends. Be well.

Acknowledgments

Ayear ago, if someone had told me I would write a book, I would have laughed. I don't write books; I read them. And I certainly don't know anything about the process. I will stay in my lane. If you would have told me how draining and difficult this past twelve-month journey would be, I would have gracefully declined, without hesitation.

During the process, I reached out to my publishing company and told them I didn't know if I could do this. I just couldn't go on. Life had come back around with a one-two punch and knocked me to the floor. How many rounds can one person take until they don't get back up? It took me a few weeks of soul-searching and a few rounds of tears, but I got back up and decided that no one knocks me down for long. What's important is getting back up every single time we are knocked down. Just keep getting back up! So I got back up, and **we finished it!**

ACKNOWLEDGMENTS

The gut-wrenching process of reliving the past nine years through my daughter's diagnosis was almost too much to endure. But I continued to hear God's encouraging words: "Don't give up." There were times when I felt as if I was having an out-of-body experience when He spoke. But He was reminding me that He never places anything on us that we cannot handle. He makes no mistakes, and His intentions are precise and accurate. So I want to thank you, God, for giving me the honor of sharing our family's story with others, and I pray that reading about our struggles will lessen theirs.

I want to thank my family for standing beside me and supporting me through this process.

Eric, thank you for sticking by my side. Although we were apart for quite some time and on different challenging journeys, know that I appreciate you and your dedication to our family.

I want to thank Madison, for allowing me to be by her side on this journey. I am so blessed I had the opportunity to stand by her and advocate with her, both for her and myself. Through this journey, there were times when she put me in my place. I would have tears streaming down my cheeks, but she set me straight: "Why are you crying?" she would ask. "You don't need to be crying." She was four years old and already an old soul for sure. She is stronger and smarter than she knows or gives herself credit for, and she continues to be a pillar of strength. Madison, I would not be the person I am today without having shared this journey with you. You truly are my *hero!* And I hope I can be yours.

ACKNOWLEDGMENTS

I also want to thank my son, Zachery, now sixteen but only six when his sister was diagnosed. He has always been such a strong person and older brother. He has a huge, gentle heart, which I admire so much. I will always feel a sting of guilt for not being able to be there for him as much as I wanted to while he was growing up, but my hope is that he has forgiven me.

I want to thank my grandmother for the cards she sent every single week! She never missed a week. Looking forward to those cards kept me going in ways she will never realize. I only wish she were here today to see Madison healthy and in such a better place than she was back when Grandma was praying for us and sending those cards.

I want to thank my writing partner, Anna Mitcheal. The story of how she and I actually came to work together was touching. I was searching for just the right person to help extract my story and met her. Anna had such a calmness about her, which actually made me uncomfortable, I think because I envied it—in her and in others who had it. It was this discomfort that ultimately pushed me to choose her as my cowriter. Anna was able to transform my broken moments, and broken memories, and into a magical story full of hope and faith. She helped me see my relationship with my parents and my brother from a different perspective, which only added to the magic of this story. The time I spent with Anna was bittersweet, and it brought healing and transformation. Although I had shed more tears during the process than I had in the past nine years, I was sad when the journey ended and Anna was on to her next project.

247

I would love to thank my editor, Jill Smith, at Forefront and the entire Forefront Books team! How I found Forefront is such a powerful story. Perhaps I will share it in my next book.